I0830812

Get A Free Book At: https://free.xspurts.com

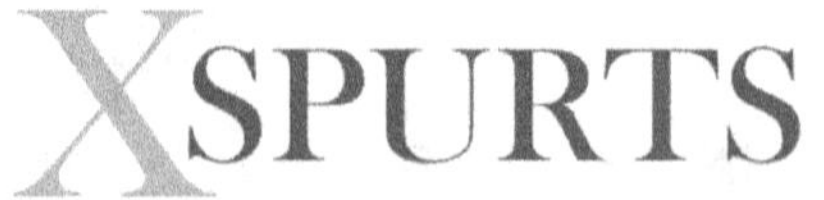

Table of Contents:

Understanding the Emotional Freedom Technique -EFT

The Emotional Freedom Technique (EFT) is a form of psychological acupressure that involves tapping on specific points on the body while focusing on emotional distress. This technique is based on the idea that negative emotions are caused by disruptions in the body's energy system, and by tapping on meridian points, a process similar to acupuncture, it helps restore balance and promote emotional healing. EFT combines elements of cognitive therapy, exposure therapy, and acupressure, making it a unique method for addressing both physical and emotional issues.

One of the key aspects of EFT is the tapping process, where individuals use their fingertips to gently tap on certain points along the body's energy meridians, typically on the face, hands, and upper body. These points correspond to energy channels in traditional Chinese medicine. As the person taps, they focus on a particular issue, allowing them to acknowledge and process the negative emotions associated with it. The process also includes verbal affirmations or statements that help reframe thoughts related to the issue being addressed.

Research into EFT's effectiveness has been growing, with many studies indicating positive outcomes for conditions such as anxiety, depression, PTSD, and chronic pain. Clinical trials have suggested that tapping can significantly reduce symptoms of stress and trauma, making it a potentially valuable tool for people struggling with emotional and physical health. For instance, a study conducted by the Association for Comprehensive Energy Psychology found that participants who used EFT experienced a significant reduction in anxiety levels, with many feeling more relaxed and balanced afterward.

Though EFT is often used for emotional well-being, it is also applied in the treatment of physical issues. Some practitioners claim that the technique can help alleviate pain, improve sleep, and even reduce the cravings associated with addictive behaviors. While these claims are still being explored through ongoing research, the widespread use of EFT by practitioners and individuals worldwide speaks to its potential efficacy.

Critics of EFT argue that it lacks the rigorous scientific foundation seen in more established psychological treatments. While EFT may not be suitable for everyone or for all conditions, many people report profound results and a sense of emotional relief after using the technique. Furthermore, because it is non-invasive and relatively simple to learn, it is a tool that individuals can use on their own, either as a complement to traditional therapy or as a stand-alone technique for emotional self-care.

As with any therapeutic method, EFT is not a one-size-fits-all solution, but its accessibility and growing body of supportive evidence suggest that it could be an effective option for many individuals seeking emotional freedom from stress, anxiety, trauma, and more.

History and development of EFT

The origins of Emotional Freedom Technique (EFT) can be traced back to the early 1990s when Gary Craig, a Stanford-trained engineer, developed the technique as a simplified version of Thought Field Therapy (TFT). TFT was created by Dr. Roger Callahan, a psychologist who, in the 1980s, began exploring the link between emotional disturbances and the body's energy system, which he believed could be influenced by stimulating specific acupressure points. Callahan's early work was groundbreaking in the field of energy psychology, and he discovered that tapping on certain points on the body could bring about profound emotional and psychological shifts.

Craig, a student of Callahan, saw the potential for improvement in TFT's complexity. TFT required practitioners to diagnose which energy meridian needed to be tapped based on the specific problem, which could make the process cumbersome. In contrast, EFT streamlined this approach by using a standardized sequence of tapping points, regardless of the issue at hand. This simplification made the technique more accessible, allowing individuals to use it for a wide range of emotional challenges without needing to be trained practitioners.

The first public mention of EFT was in 1995, when Gary Craig released a free manual detailing the technique. The manual explained how tapping on specific meridian points while focusing on an emotional problem could release blockages and lead to emotional healing. Craig's open-access approach contributed to the technique's rapid spread, as it allowed people around the world to experiment with EFT on their own. Within a few years, EFT began gaining recognition from both practitioners and individuals who experienced personal success with the method.

EFT's growing popularity was further bolstered by its integration into the broader field of energy psychology, which combines elements of traditional Chinese medicine, acupressure, and cognitive therapy. The rise of the internet in the late 1990s and early 2000s helped spread EFT worldwide. Online resources, forums, and videos made it easier for people to learn the technique, share their experiences, and find support in using EFT for various issues like stress, anxiety, trauma, and even physical pain.

In the early 2000s, research into the effectiveness of EFT began to emerge. Studies on EFT's impact on stress reduction, emotional well-being, and chronic pain have steadily increased, with some showing positive results. One of the most significant studies was conducted in 2012 by Dr. Dawson Church, a leading researcher in the field of energy psychology, which found that EFT could lower cortisol levels (the stress hormone) and provide lasting emotional benefits. This type of research helped to establish EFT as a legitimate tool in the world of alternative healing and psychology.

While EFT was initially met with skepticism from some psychologists and medical professionals, its simplicity and accessibility have contributed to its widespread acceptance among people seeking alternative therapies. Today, EFT is practiced by thousands of individuals worldwide, from licensed therapists to laypeople who use it for self-help. It has expanded beyond its initial focus on emotional distress to include areas such as pain management, performance enhancement, and personal growth.

The continued evolution of EFT includes the development of specialized variations, such as Matrix Reimprinting, which focuses on transforming traumatic memories, and the use of EFT in conjunction with other therapeutic modalities, such as hypnosis and coaching. As EFT grows in both research and application, it remains an innovative and accessible approach to emotional and psychological healing, deeply rooted in the belief that the mind and body are intricately connected.

Principles of EFT

The principles behind Emotional Freedom Technique (EFT) are grounded in the belief that emotional and physical well-being are closely connected to the flow of energy within the body. According to this framework, negative emotions, stress, and trauma are the result of blockages or imbalances in the body's energy system. By tapping on specific acupressure points while focusing on an emotional issue, EFT aims to clear these disruptions, restore balance, and promote healing.

One of the core principles of EFT is the concept of "psychological reversal," which suggests that when negative emotions or unresolved trauma are present, the body's energy system becomes disrupted, creating internal resistance to healing. EFT addresses this by helping individuals release emotional blockages, allowing energy to flow freely and fostering a sense of emotional freedom. This process involves tapping on meridian points, which are energy pathways that have been mapped in traditional Chinese medicine. Each meridian is associated with a specific area of the body and is thought to influence different emotions, behaviors, or physiological responses.

Another fundamental principle of EFT is the mind-body connection. EFT posits that unresolved emotional issues can manifest as physical symptoms, including pain, tension, or fatigue. By targeting the underlying emotional causes of these physical issues, EFT seeks to alleviate both emotional and physical distress. For example, someone dealing with anxiety might experience a racing heart, shortness of breath, or tight muscles. By tapping on specific points while focusing on the anxiety, EFT aims to reduce both the emotional response and the physical symptoms, promoting an overall sense of relaxation.

The process of tapping itself is integral to EFT's principles. Tapping involves lightly tapping with the fingertips on specific meridian points, often starting from the top of the head and moving down the body to the chest and hands. This action is thought to stimulate the energy system, allowing for the release of negative emotions. The combination of physical tapping and focused attention on the issue at hand helps to desensitize the emotional response, reducing its intensity over time. This process is often referred to as "tuning" the energy system.

EFT also emphasizes the importance of self-awareness and emotional acceptance. A key principle of EFT is the need for individuals to fully acknowledge and accept their emotional experiences, rather than suppressing or avoiding them. In fact, during an EFT session, individuals are encouraged to identify and verbally express the negative emotion they are experiencing (e.g., fear, anger, sadness) while tapping on the meridian points. This act of acknowledgment and acceptance is thought to reduce the emotional charge associated with the issue, facilitating emotional release and healing.

Additionally, EFT incorporates the idea of "global statements" and "specific statements" when working through emotional issues. A global statement might address a general feeling or emotional state, such as "Even though I feel anxious, I deeply and completely accept myself." Specific statements, on the other hand, focus on particular aspects of the issue, such as "Even though I feel afraid of public speaking, I accept this fear." The balance of both types of statements helps individuals address both the broad emotional challenge and the specific aspects of the issue they are trying to heal.

The principle of working with both the conscious and unconscious mind is also essential to EFT. It recognizes that emotional blockages may exist on both conscious and unconscious levels. Through tapping, EFT is thought to help individuals access deeper emotional layers, allowing them to process and release unresolved issues that may not be immediately apparent. This principle underlines EFT's holistic approach, addressing both the surface-level and underlying causes of emotional distress.

Lastly, the principle of self-empowerment is central to EFT. One of the key advantages of this technique is that it is accessible for self-use. While practitioners can guide individuals through the tapping process, EFT can also be performed independently, giving individuals the tools to manage their emotions and promote healing on their own terms. This self-reliance is empowering for those seeking to take control of their emotional health, offering a practical method for emotional regulation and personal growth.

By combining these principles — energy system balancing, mind-body connection, emotional acceptance, and self-empowerment — EFT provides a unique approach to emotional healing. It offers a versatile and accessible method for addressing a wide range of emotional challenges, from stress and anxiety to trauma and phobias, making it a valuable tool in both therapeutic settings and for self-care.

Core elements of EFT practice

The practice of Emotional Freedom Technique (EFT) revolves around several core elements that combine psychological principles, physical tapping, and focused intention to promote emotional healing. These elements work together to address both the emotional and physical aspects of distress, allowing individuals to manage negative feelings, alleviate stress, and restore balance within the body's energy system.

The first core element is the **identification of the issue**. EFT begins with the individual identifying a specific emotional or physical problem they wish to address. This could be anything from anxiety or fear to chronic pain or past trauma. Clearly defining the issue is crucial because it helps the person focus their attention and intention on the precise emotional disturbance they want to clear. The clarity of the problem is important because it allows for a more targeted and effective tapping process.

The second core element is the **setup statement**. This is a phrase or affirmation used during the initial phase of EFT, designed to acknowledge and accept the emotional issue without judgment. Typically, the setup statement follows a structure like, "Even though I have this [issue], I deeply and completely accept myself." The setup statement helps to neutralize the emotional charge surrounding the problem and creates a sense of self-compassion. It also allows individuals to emotionally accept their feelings, which is a key part of the healing process.

The third key element is the **tapping sequence**. EFT involves tapping on a series of specific acupressure points on the body, usually with the fingertips. These points are located along the body's energy meridians, which are pathways through which vital energy flows, according to traditional Chinese medicine. The sequence typically starts with the **karate chop point** (on the side of the hand), followed by tapping on key points such as the top of the head, the eyebrows, the sides of the eyes, under the eyes, under the nose, the chin, the collarbone, and under the arms. Each point corresponds to a different energy pathway, and tapping on them is believed to stimulate the energy system, releasing blockages and restoring balance.

Another crucial element is **focus on the emotional issue**. As the individual taps on the meridian points, they simultaneously focus on the specific problem they are addressing. This might involve thinking about the intensity of the negative emotion, recalling a traumatic memory, or simply feeling the physical discomfort associated with the issue. The idea is that by tapping while focused on the problem, the individual allows the body's energy system to reprocess and release the emotional charge tied to the issue. This process is often referred to as "desensitizing" the emotional intensity of the problem.

The **rating of emotional intensity** is another core element in EFT practice. Before starting the tapping process, individuals typically rate the intensity of their emotional distress on a scale from 0 to 10, with 0 being no distress and 10 being the highest level of emotional disturbance. This rating provides a benchmark for measuring progress during the session. As the tapping process unfolds, individuals reassess their emotional intensity after each round of tapping. A decrease in the rating indicates that the tapping has had a positive effect in reducing the emotional charge linked to the issue.

Following the tapping sequence, **re-evaluation** of the emotional issue takes place. After several rounds of tapping, individuals check back in with their emotions to see how they feel. If the emotional intensity has decreased significantly, the process is considered successful. If the intensity remains high, further rounds of tapping or modifications to the setup statement may be necessary. Some practitioners suggest tapping on related aspects or adopting a different angle to explore the issue more deeply.

Finally, a core element of EFT is **self-empowerment**. One of the main advantages of EFT is that it is a self-administered technique, which means individuals can use it independently for personal growth, emotional regulation, or to address everyday stress. Practitioners and individuals alike often report that EFT offers a sense of control over their emotional well-being, allowing them to address feelings of anxiety, fear, and other negative emotions as they arise, without the need for expensive or time-consuming treatments.

In addition to these core elements, EFT is flexible and adaptable, making it accessible for a wide range of issues, from anxiety and depression to pain management and performance enhancement. The combination of focused tapping, emotional acceptance, and self-awareness forms the foundation of EFT practice, empowering individuals to achieve emotional freedom and cultivate a greater sense of well-being.

Learning the EFT Tapping Techniques

Learning the Emotional Freedom Technique (EFT) tapping techniques involves understanding a series of simple steps that combine mental focus, emotional awareness, and physical tapping on key meridian points. By tapping on specific acupressure points while concentrating on a particular issue, individuals can release negative emotions, reduce stress, and achieve greater emotional balance. The process is straightforward, but like any skill, it requires practice and self-awareness to be most effective.

The first step in learning EFT is to **identify the issue** that you want to address. This can be an emotional challenge, such as anxiety, fear, or sadness, or a physical issue like pain or tension. It's important to be specific about the problem, as EFT works best when you are clear and focused on a single issue at a time. This allows the energy system to target the root of the problem rather than trying to solve multiple issues simultaneously.

Once the issue is identified, the next step is to **rate the intensity** of the emotion or discomfort on a scale from 0 to 10. This rating serves as a benchmark, helping you measure your progress throughout the tapping process. The higher the number, the more intense the emotional or physical reaction to the issue. After tapping, you will re-rate the intensity to see how much it has decreased.

The central action of EFT involves **tapping on specific acupressure points**. These points, which are based on energy meridians in traditional Chinese medicine, are thought to correspond to different aspects of the body's energy flow. The standard tapping sequence starts with the **karate chop point** on the side of the hand, which is used to set the intention and acknowledge the issue. This is followed by tapping on the top of the head, the eyebrow, the side of the eye, under the eye, under the nose, the chin, the collarbone, and under the arms. Each point is tapped gently with the fingertips while focusing on the issue you wish to address.

During the tapping sequence, it's important to **repeat a setup statement**. The setup statement is a positive affirmation that combines emotional acknowledgment with self-acceptance. For example, if you're addressing anxiety, the setup statement might be, "Even though I feel anxious about this situation, I deeply and completely accept myself." Repeating this statement while tapping on the karate chop point helps to neutralize the emotional charge associated with the issue, promoting emotional acceptance and reducing resistance.

As you tap through the sequence, it's essential to **focus on the emotional or physical discomfort** tied to the issue. You may think about the feelings or the situation that caused the distress, or you can simply focus on the sensations in your body. For example, if you feel tightness in your chest when thinking about a stressful situation, you can focus on that physical sensation as you tap. The tapping itself is thought to signal the body's energy system to release these emotional blockages, reducing the intensity of the feelings over time.

Throughout the process, you can also incorporate **reminder phrases** that help keep your attention on the issue. These are short statements or words that you repeat as you tap. For example, you might say, "This anxiety," or "The fear of failure," as you tap through each point. These reminders reinforce your focus on the problem, helping the energy system clear the emotional blockages more effectively.

After completing one round of tapping, it's important to **re-assess the intensity** of the issue. On a scale from 0 to 10, how much has the emotional intensity decreased? If the intensity has gone down significantly, that's a sign that the tapping has been effective. However, if the intensity is still high, you may need to continue tapping or address another aspect of the issue. It's not unusual to need multiple rounds of tapping to fully clear a particularly stubborn emotion or issue.

The **self-empowerment** aspect of EFT is also a key factor in learning and using the technique. Once you understand the basic principles and steps, EFT becomes a tool you can use anytime to manage stress, relieve anxiety, or address other emotional challenges. This independence can be especially helpful for people who experience overwhelming emotions or want to take control of their emotional well-being in everyday situations.

In addition to the basic tapping sequence, EFT practitioners often recommend **tailoring the approach** for different types of emotional issues. For example, if a person is dealing with trauma or deep-seated fears, they may need to break down the issue into smaller, more specific aspects and tap on them separately. Some people also incorporate **visualization** techniques, imagining the problem or memory dissolving as they tap, or they might use **positive affirmations** to replace negative beliefs with healthier ones.

Lastly, it's important to **practice regularly**. Like any skill, the more you practice EFT, the more effective it becomes. Consistent use can lead to greater emotional resilience, reduced stress, and improved overall well-being. Many people find that using EFT regularly helps them maintain a sense of calm and balance in their lives, making it a powerful tool for emotional self-care.

Learning EFT tapping techniques offers a simple yet effective way to address emotional issues, reduce stress, and restore energy balance. With practice and attention, this method can provide lasting benefits for anyone seeking a holistic approach to emotional healing and personal growth.

The basics of Emotional Freedom Technique (EFT) tapping are centered around a straightforward, yet powerful approach to emotional and physical healing. At its core, EFT involves tapping on specific acupressure points on the body while focusing on a particular issue or emotional discomfort. This combination of tapping and mindful attention aims to release blockages in the body's energy system, which are believed to cause negative emotions and physical distress.

The tapping process begins with the **identification of the issue**. Whether it's an emotion like anxiety, fear, or anger, or a physical symptom such as pain or tension, identifying the exact issue you want to address is key to the technique's success. It's important to be specific about the problem, as focusing on one issue at a time allows for more effective energy clearing.

Once the issue is defined, the next step is to create a **setup statement**, which is an affirmation used to acknowledge and accept the issue at hand. The setup statement typically follows a format like: "Even though I feel [emotion or issue], I deeply and completely accept myself." This statement helps to neutralize the emotional charge related to the issue, setting the intention for healing. It is repeated while tapping on the **karate chop point**, located on the side of the hand.

Next, the individual proceeds to the **tapping sequence**, which involves gently tapping on a series of meridian points along the body. These meridian points are located on energy pathways used in traditional Chinese medicine and are thought to correspond to different emotions and physical sensations. The typical tapping sequence begins at the **karate chop point** and then moves to the following locations:

- **Top of the head** (crown)
- **Eyebrow** (near the bridge of the nose)
- **Side of the eye** (at the temple)
- **Under the eye** (on the cheekbone)
- **Under the nose** (between the nose and upper lip)
- **Chin** (in the crease between the chin and lower lip)
- **Collarbone** (just below the collarbone)
- **Under the arm** (about 4 inches below the armpit)

Each point is tapped lightly with the fingertips about 5-7 times while focusing on the issue at hand. The tapping stimulates the body's energy system, facilitating the release of negative emotions and restoring balance.

Throughout the tapping process, it's important to **focus on the emotional or physical sensations** linked to the issue. This could mean thinking about a specific stressful event or simply noticing how the body feels when experiencing discomfort. The key is to stay present with the feelings, as this enhances the effectiveness of the tapping in clearing out emotional blockages.

As the tapping sequence progresses, it's helpful to **re-rate the intensity** of the emotional or physical discomfort on a scale of 0 to 10, with 0 representing no distress and 10 representing the highest intensity. After a few rounds of tapping, individuals reassess the intensity to determine whether there has been a decrease. If the intensity has dropped, it indicates that the tapping is working to reduce the emotional charge tied to the issue.

Another basic concept in EFT is the use of **reminder phrases**. These are brief phrases or keywords that help keep focus on the problem while tapping. For example, someone working on a fear of public speaking might use a reminder phrase like, "This fear of speaking" while tapping through the points. These reminder phrases keep the mind focused on the specific issue being worked on, helping to clear it more effectively.

The ultimate goal of EFT is to **achieve emotional release**. As the body's energy system becomes unblocked, the negative emotions tied to a particular event or issue are expected to diminish in intensity. This often leads to a feeling of lightness, calm, and emotional relief. Many people find that after a few sessions, they feel more relaxed, centered, and better equipped to handle stress or emotional challenges.

In addition to emotional issues, EFT is also used for a variety of physical symptoms, such as chronic pain, tension, or sleep disturbances. The belief is that unresolved emotions can contribute to physical problems, and by tapping to release these emotional blockages, physical symptoms can improve or even dissipate.

Learning the basics of EFT tapping is accessible to anyone and can be done on your own or with the help of a trained practitioner. It's a versatile technique that can be used for a wide range of issues, from anxiety and trauma to everyday stress. As a self-help tool, EFT empowers individuals to take charge of their emotional well-being, offering a simple, non-invasive way to promote healing and balance.

Advanced tapping techniques

Advanced Emotional Freedom Technique (EFT) tapping techniques build upon the basic principles of EFT but incorporate more nuanced approaches to address deeper emotional issues, complex trauma, or persistent physical symptoms. These techniques allow practitioners to tailor the EFT process to specific challenges, enabling more profound and lasting results.

One of the most widely used advanced techniques is **the Movie Technique**. This approach is particularly helpful when working with trauma or distressing memories. The individual visualizes the troubling memory, as if watching it like a movie. As they tap through the meridian points, they observe the memory from a detached, neutral perspective. This method helps reduce the emotional charge associated with the memory, enabling the person to process it without becoming overwhelmed by the feelings attached to it. By repeatedly tapping on the meridian points while focusing on the memory, the person can desensitize themselves to the emotional intensity of the event.

Another powerful advanced technique is **the Tell the Story Method**. This involves fully recounting the traumatic or emotionally charged event while tapping. As the person speaks about the event, they remain focused on the feelings that arise during the storytelling process. This method helps to release any pent-up emotions connected to the story and can bring relief to those holding onto repressed memories or feelings. The act of verbalizing the experience while tapping on the points allows for emotional release and greater understanding of how the issue has been impacting the individual's life.

Chasing the Pain is an advanced technique often used for physical symptoms or chronic pain. It works by identifying the specific area of pain in the body and using tapping to focus on that sensation. As the person taps, they may notice the pain shifting or moving to different parts of the body. EFT practitioners call this "chasing the pain," and the process helps individuals identify and release the emotional components tied to their physical discomfort. This technique can help people with chronic conditions, as emotional blocks often contribute to persistent physical pain.

Matrix Reimprinting is another advanced EFT technique that combines elements of EFT with visualization and inner child work. Developed by Karl Dawson, this method allows individuals to tap into past memories and re-imprint them with positive emotions. The process involves imagining oneself as a child in a past event and then "rewriting" that memory while tapping. By re-imprinting the memory with new, more empowering beliefs, individuals can heal the emotional wounds associated with that event, shifting their perception and emotional response to it. This technique is especially helpful for those with deep-seated trauma or limiting beliefs formed in childhood.

For those dealing with **self-sabotage** or deeply ingrained negative patterns, the **EFT Choices Method** can be effective. This technique works by helping the individual acknowledge the negative belief or behavior pattern and then "swap" it for a healthier, more empowering alternative. During the tapping process, the person taps while holding the intention to replace the old belief with a new one. For example, if someone is tapping to release the belief "I'm not good enough," they would also tap on the new belief, "I am worthy and capable." This creates a shift in mindset and helps reprogram the subconscious mind to support more positive behaviors and beliefs.

The Personal Peace Procedure is a comprehensive advanced technique designed to address a wide range of emotional issues. It involves tapping on various past memories, experiences, and traumas, working systematically through any unresolved emotional challenges. Individuals start by identifying specific memories, rating their emotional intensity, and tapping through each one. This procedure can help people clear long-standing emotional baggage and create a deeper sense of peace and emotional freedom. It's often recommended as a method for those who want to tackle multiple emotional issues in a holistic way.

In **EFT for Performance Enhancement**, advanced techniques focus on removing blocks related to performance anxiety, lack of confidence, or limiting beliefs in specific areas such as sports, public speaking, or creative endeavors. The person taps while visualizing the desired performance or outcome, such as giving a successful speech or achieving a personal best in a sport. The tapping helps to release fears or doubts that may prevent them from achieving their goals, allowing for improved focus, confidence, and performance.

Lastly, **EFT with affirmation reframing** is a technique where tapping is combined with positive affirmations that are personalized for the individual's specific situation. Instead of just tapping through negative emotions, the person incorporates statements like, "I am confident," "I trust myself," or "I am in control," reinforcing positive beliefs during the tapping process. This combination of releasing negative emotions while reinforcing positive ones can help to rewire the subconscious mind, creating lasting changes in behavior and emotional state.

Advanced EFT techniques provide powerful tools for deep emotional healing and personal transformation. Whether addressing trauma, chronic pain, performance anxiety, or limiting beliefs, these techniques offer ways to access deeper layers of the psyche and release long-held emotional blockages. As practitioners become more familiar with these methods, they can tailor EFT to more effectively treat complex and persistent issues, making it an even more versatile and profound therapeutic approach.

The EFT Tapping Sequence

The EFT tapping sequence is a fundamental process that combines gentle tapping on specific acupressure points with focused mental attention to address emotional and physical distress. This sequence is based on the principles of traditional Chinese medicine, which identifies energy meridians throughout the body. By tapping on these key points, EFT is believed to clear blockages in the body's energy system, restoring emotional balance and promoting healing.

The tapping sequence begins with the **setup statement**, a crucial part of the process. This statement is a way of acknowledging the issue at hand while accepting oneself despite the discomfort. Typically, the setup is done by tapping on the **karate chop point**, located on the side of the hand. The setup statement might look something like, "Even though I feel [emotion or issue], I deeply and completely accept myself." This helps to reduce resistance and opens the energy system for healing.

Once the setup statement is completed, the practitioner moves on to the tapping sequence. The basic sequence follows a specific order of meridian points, starting at the top of the head and working down the body. Here are the key tapping points and their locations:

1. **Top of the Head (Crown)**: Tap gently on the crown of the head, which is thought to connect to the body's energy field and overall well-being.
2. **Eyebrow**: At the beginning of the eyebrow, where it meets the bridge of the nose, tap lightly on this point to address issues tied to deep thought or mental clarity.
3. **Side of the Eye**: Located at the outer edge of the eye socket, this point is believed to help release emotions linked to stress, fear, or unresolved thoughts.
4. **Under the Eye**: Tap just below the eye, on the bone, to address feelings of fear, anxiety, or discomfort related to self-image or past trauma.
5. **Under the Nose**: Tap just beneath the nose, in the area between the nose and upper lip, which is thought to help release suppressed feelings or unresolved issues.
6. **Chin**: Tap on the small indentation between the chin and lower lip, targeting emotional issues that may be linked to communication or self-expression.
7. **Collarbone**: Tap on the soft spot just below the collarbone, which is associated with addressing stress, overwhelm, and feelings of being "stuck."
8. **Under the Arm**: About four inches below the armpit, this point is often tapped to release emotional blocks related to fear, anxiety, and unresolved trauma.

Throughout the sequence, it's important to focus on the emotional or physical issue you're addressing. While tapping, repeat **reminder phrases** to keep the focus on the specific problem, such as, "This fear of flying" or "This anxiety about work." These phrases help reinforce the focus on the issue while activating the body's energy system.

After completing the first round of tapping, individuals are encouraged to reassess the emotional intensity of the issue on a scale of 0 to 10. If the intensity has decreased, the process is typically repeated, with the intensity rating often lowering with each round. Sometimes, adjustments to the setup statement or reminder phrase may be needed if the emotional charge persists.

The sequence can be repeated multiple times until the emotional or physical issue has diminished in intensity. Once a significant reduction is achieved, a final round may involve tapping with **positive affirmations**. For example, after addressing an issue like anxiety, the person might tap with affirmations such as, "I am calm and in control," or "I trust myself and feel at peace." This helps reinforce the new, positive emotional state and strengthens the changes made during the tapping process.

The beauty of the EFT tapping sequence is its simplicity and versatility. Whether used to reduce stress, alleviate anxiety, or address physical pain, this sequence allows individuals to take control of their emotional and physical well-being. With practice, it becomes an easy, accessible tool that can be used anytime to restore emotional balance and clear blocked energy.

The Science behind EFT

The science behind Emotional Freedom Technique (EFT) draws from several established fields, including energy psychology, neuroscience, and acupressure. Though the technique remains somewhat controversial in traditional medical circles, a growing body of research supports its effectiveness in addressing emotional and physical issues. The core idea is that EFT taps into the body's energy system to release blockages that may contribute to emotional distress and physical ailments.

At the heart of EFT is the concept of **energy meridians**, a core element of Traditional Chinese Medicine (TCM). According to TCM, the body has a network of energy pathways through which life force, or "Qi" (pronounced "chee"), flows. When these pathways are blocked or disrupted, it is believed that physical or emotional issues can arise. The meridian points used in EFT correspond to these pathways, and tapping on them is thought to stimulate energy flow, helping to restore balance and alleviate distress.

Research into **psychoneuroimmunology** (PNI) provides a framework for understanding how emotions can affect the body's physical health. PNI studies how psychological factors influence the nervous and immune systems. Negative emotions such as stress, fear, or trauma can activate the body's "fight or flight" response, triggering the release of stress hormones like cortisol. Over time, chronic stress can weaken the immune system, contribute to inflammation, and exacerbate conditions like anxiety, depression, or chronic pain. EFT is thought to help regulate these stress responses by tapping into the energy system, calming the autonomic nervous system, and reducing the physiological effects of stress.

Several studies have explored the impact of EFT on the brain, particularly in the context of **neuroplasticity**—the brain's ability to rewire itself in response to new experiences. When individuals experience intense emotional trauma or chronic stress, their brain patterns can become "wired" to respond in ways that perpetuate those negative emotional states. EFT may help break these neural patterns by promoting relaxation and encouraging the brain to form new, more balanced associations. Functional Magnetic Resonance Imaging (fMRI) and Electroencephalography (EEG) studies have shown changes in brain activity after EFT sessions, indicating that the technique may help re-regulate brain function and reduce emotional reactivity.

EFT also aligns with **theories of acupuncture and acupressure**, where stimulating certain points on the body is believed to restore balance to the energy system. While traditional acupuncture uses needles, EFT uses tapping to stimulate the same meridian points. This physical stimulation is thought to activate the body's natural healing processes, reduce tension, and help clear blockages in the energy system. The tapping may also trigger the release of **endorphins**, the body's natural "feel-good" chemicals, which contribute to a sense of relaxation and emotional well-being.

The **stress-reducing effects** of EFT are particularly well-documented in clinical research. In studies comparing EFT with other stress-reduction techniques, such as cognitive behavioral therapy (CBT) or mindfulness, EFT has shown comparable or superior results in reducing anxiety, stress, and emotional distress. For example, research published in the *Journal of Nervous and Mental Disease* found that participants who used EFT experienced a significant reduction in anxiety levels after just one session, and the benefits were sustained over time. Similarly, a study in the *Journal of Clinical Psychology* showed that EFT significantly reduced PTSD symptoms in veterans, suggesting its potential for treating trauma.

Further, the **biochemical changes** associated with EFT provide additional evidence of its effectiveness. Studies have found that EFT reduces cortisol levels, a key indicator of stress, in individuals who experience chronic anxiety. In one study, participants' cortisol levels were measured before and after an EFT session, and the results showed a marked reduction in cortisol, indicating that EFT helped to alleviate stress and emotional tension at a biochemical level.

EFT's effectiveness may also be linked to **the placebo effect**, where belief in the healing process itself contributes to improvement. However, while placebo effects are common in many healing practices, research has shown that EFT produces real, measurable changes in brain and body function, suggesting that the technique is more than just a mind-over-matter phenomenon.

The combination of **psychological, physiological, and energetic principles** makes EFT a holistic treatment option. While more research is needed to fully understand the underlying mechanisms, the existing body of evidence suggests that EFT may have a powerful impact on emotional regulation, stress management, and physical health. By tapping on acupressure points while focusing on an issue, EFT appears to help release emotional blockages, restore balance in the body's energy system, and bring about lasting changes in emotional and physical well-being. As science continues to explore the connections between mind, body, and energy, EFT stands as a promising tool for both self-care and therapeutic intervention.

The psychological and emotional aspects of Emotional Freedom Technique (EFT) are central to its effectiveness in addressing a wide range of mental and emotional issues. EFT combines principles from cognitive psychology and acupressure to provide a holistic approach to healing, focusing on the emotional roots of distress. By tapping on specific acupressure points while concentrating on a problem or negative emotion, individuals can bring awareness to their emotional states and facilitate a process of emotional release and healing.

One of the core psychological concepts behind EFT is the idea that **unresolved emotional issues** create blockages in the body's energy system. These emotional blockages are thought to manifest as psychological distress or physical symptoms, such as anxiety, depression, or chronic pain. EFT works by targeting the emotional experience directly—allowing individuals to confront negative emotions without the need for verbal expression or intense confrontation. As the person taps on the meridian points, the energy flow is thought to be restored, which helps reduce the intensity of the emotion and promote healing.

Emotional regulation is another key aspect of EFT. Many individuals struggle with emotional dysregulation, where emotions become overwhelming or difficult to manage. This often occurs when the brain's emotional response system is activated by stress, trauma, or unprocessed feelings. By using EFT, individuals can bring these emotions into their conscious awareness, allowing them to reframe the emotional experience. The tapping process itself has a calming effect, reducing the intensity of negative emotions like fear, anger, or sadness. This calming effect helps individuals regain control over their emotional responses, making it easier to handle difficult situations in a balanced way.

EFT is particularly effective in addressing **trauma and past emotional wounds**. Whether it's childhood trauma, a past abusive relationship, or an event that caused long-term emotional pain, EFT allows individuals to revisit these painful memories and neutralize the emotional charge tied to them. Unlike traditional talk therapy, which may involve lengthy discussion or analysis of the trauma, EFT provides a more direct, embodied approach. Through tapping, individuals can process the emotional aspects of the trauma without becoming overwhelmed by the memory or reliving the pain. This can make the healing process faster and less distressing.

Belief systems also play a significant role in emotional and psychological well-being. Many negative emotions are linked to limiting beliefs or distorted thought patterns, such as "I'm not good enough," "I'll never succeed," or "I don't deserve love." These beliefs can create a negative feedback loop, reinforcing feelings of anxiety, depression, or self-doubt. EFT addresses these beliefs by helping individuals acknowledge and challenge them, replacing them with healthier, more empowering thoughts. By tapping while focusing on these negative beliefs, individuals can begin to weaken the emotional charge they carry and replace them with positive affirmations, leading to a shift in mindset and emotional state.

The **mind-body connection** is another important factor in the psychological and emotional benefits of EFT. Research has shown that emotions are often experienced physically, with certain feelings manifesting as tension, pain, or discomfort in specific areas of the body. For example, stress might show up as tightness in the chest, while anxiety could manifest as a stomach ache. EFT works directly with this mind-body connection by focusing on the physical sensations associated with emotional issues. By tapping on the acupressure points while tuning into the physical sensations, individuals can clear these physical manifestations of emotional distress, leading to both emotional relief and physical relaxation.

Self-awareness and mindfulness are integral to the process of EFT. The technique encourages individuals to pay close attention to their thoughts, feelings, and bodily sensations. This heightened self-awareness is essential for identifying the underlying emotional issues that need to be addressed. By becoming more mindful of the emotional and physical cues that arise during tapping, individuals can gain greater insight into their emotional patterns and how they react to certain triggers. This increased awareness can be empowering, helping individuals take a more active role in their emotional health and well-being.

Another psychological benefit of EFT is its ability to **reduce stress and anxiety**. The technique has been shown to lower cortisol levels, the body's primary stress hormone, making it a valuable tool for managing chronic stress. Stress, when left unchecked, can lead to a host of psychological issues, including anxiety, depression, and burnout. EFT helps break the cycle of stress by promoting relaxation, providing individuals with a tool they can use to calm their minds and bodies in moments of distress.

The emotional healing that EFT facilitates is not just about symptom relief but also about **emotional empowerment**. As individuals work through their emotional issues using EFT, they gain a sense of control over their feelings. Rather than being at the mercy of overwhelming emotions or negative thought patterns, they learn to address emotional challenges in a constructive way. This empowerment extends to other areas of life, allowing individuals to approach relationships, work, and personal goals with greater emotional resilience.

In essence, the psychological and emotional aspects of EFT revolve around the concept of energy balance—clearing blockages, releasing trapped emotions, and restoring a sense of emotional freedom. By combining physical tapping with mental and emotional awareness, EFT provides a powerful tool for individuals to heal emotional wounds, regulate their emotions, and cultivate a more positive emotional state. Whether used for everyday stress management or to address deep-seated trauma, EFT offers a pathway to emotional well-being that is both effective and empowering.

The physical and physiological aspects of Emotional Freedom Technique (EFT) are deeply intertwined with the body's energy system and the ways in which emotions manifest physically. At the core of EFT is the idea that emotional distress, when left unresolved, can create blockages in the body's energy pathways, leading to physical symptoms such as pain, tension, or illness. By tapping on specific acupressure points along these energy pathways, EFT is believed to release these blockages, promoting physical healing and emotional balance.

One of the primary physical benefits of EFT is its ability to **reduce stress**. When the body experiences stress, it activates the autonomic nervous system, triggering the "fight or flight" response. This leads to an increase in the production of stress hormones, particularly cortisol and adrenaline, which prepare the body to react to a perceived threat. While this response is beneficial in short bursts, chronic stress can lead to negative physiological outcomes, such as elevated blood pressure, weakened immune function, and digestive issues. EFT has been shown to lower cortisol levels, helping to counteract the physical effects of stress. By tapping on acupressure points while focusing on a stressful issue, individuals can calm their nervous system, reduce the physiological markers of stress, and restore balance to the body's systems.

EFT's impact on the **immune system** is another area of interest. Chronic emotional distress and high levels of stress can weaken the immune system, making the body more susceptible to illness. High cortisol levels can suppress the immune system, reducing the body's ability to fight infections and repair tissue damage. Several studies have shown that EFT can improve immune functioning by lowering cortisol and promoting relaxation. As the body's stress response is alleviated, immune system activity is enhanced, which may improve overall health and resilience.

In addition to stress and immunity, EFT can also have a direct impact on **pain management**. Many people use EFT to address chronic pain, which is often exacerbated by emotional factors. Studies have shown that emotional and psychological stress can intensify pain perception, and addressing the emotional components of pain can lead to significant relief. By tapping on specific meridian points while focusing on the pain, EFT can help reduce the emotional intensity associated with the physical sensation, making the pain more manageable. This reduction in emotional distress may also result in a decrease in muscle tension, which is often a contributing factor to pain in areas like the back, neck, or shoulders.

Muscle relaxation is another key physiological benefit of EFT. When the body experiences emotional stress, it tends to hold tension in various muscle groups. This tension can lead to headaches, jaw pain, back pain, and other physical discomforts. By using EFT, individuals can activate the parasympathetic nervous system, which is responsible for the "rest and digest" response. This system helps to relax the muscles, reduce blood pressure, and lower heart rate, promoting a state of calm and physical relaxation. As the body releases this tension, individuals may experience greater flexibility, less discomfort, and an overall sense of physical well-being.

EFT has also been found to have a positive effect on **sleep**. Stress, anxiety, and unresolved emotions are often contributors to poor sleep quality. By reducing the body's stress response and promoting emotional regulation, EFT can help individuals achieve better, more restful sleep. Studies have shown that individuals who practice EFT regularly experience fewer sleep disturbances, reduced anxiety before bed, and a greater sense of relaxation when trying to fall asleep. The physiological relaxation induced by EFT may help reduce the physical discomfort that can interfere with sleep, allowing individuals to rest more deeply.

The **cardiovascular system** is another area where EFT may have a beneficial impact. Chronic stress is known to contribute to increased blood pressure, higher heart rates, and greater strain on the cardiovascular system. By promoting a relaxation response and lowering cortisol levels, EFT can help mitigate these effects. In fact, research has shown that EFT can lead to a reduction in both systolic and diastolic blood pressure, as well as heart rate, when individuals focus on a stressful situation or emotion while tapping. This makes EFT a useful tool for managing conditions such as hypertension and cardiovascular stress.

One of the most remarkable aspects of EFT is its ability to address the **psychosomatic connection**, where emotional distress manifests as physical symptoms. This connection is particularly evident in conditions like fibromyalgia, irritable bowel syndrome (IBS), and tension headaches, where physical symptoms are often exacerbated by emotional triggers. EFT helps by targeting the emotional root cause of these conditions, addressing the mental and emotional factors that contribute to the physical discomfort. By releasing emotional tension through tapping, individuals may experience a reduction in both emotional distress and physical symptoms, improving their overall health and quality of life.

Additionally, EFT can promote **neurological balance**. Emotional experiences often cause changes in brain activity, particularly in areas related to stress and emotional regulation, such as the amygdala and prefrontal cortex. Research has shown that EFT can affect brain activity, helping to reduce the activation of the amygdala (which plays a role in fear and stress) and promote greater regulation by the prefrontal cortex. This may explain the calming effect of EFT, as well as its ability to reduce emotional reactivity and improve cognitive function. The balance achieved through EFT may help individuals process emotions more effectively, reducing the physiological toll of unresolved emotions.

Overall, the physical and physiological benefits of EFT are vast and multifaceted. By addressing emotional blockages and stress, EFT has the potential to improve physical health by promoting relaxation, reducing pain, enhancing immune function, and improving sleep. As research continues to explore the physiological mechanisms of EFT, it becomes increasingly clear that the practice offers a holistic approach to health, bridging the gap between the mind and body for a more balanced and harmonious state of well-being.

Recent studies and scientific evidence

Recent studies and scientific evidence have increasingly supported the effectiveness of Emotional Freedom Technique (EFT) in addressing a variety of psychological and physical issues. Research has shown that EFT can significantly reduce stress, anxiety, depression, and PTSD symptoms, while also offering benefits for pain management and overall emotional well-being. Much of this research focuses on the physiological and neurological changes that occur during EFT sessions, providing insight into how the technique works at the biological level.

One of the most compelling areas of research involves **EFT's impact on stress and cortisol levels**. Cortisol, the body's primary stress hormone, is known to play a key role in the physical effects of stress, including immune suppression and inflammation. A study published in the *Journal of Nervous and Mental Disease* found that individuals who participated in EFT sessions experienced a significant reduction in cortisol levels. The research indicated that a single session of EFT could reduce cortisol by up to 43%, suggesting that the technique can help regulate the body's stress response in a measurable and immediate way.

Studies have also demonstrated EFT's effectiveness in treating **anxiety and PTSD**. In a randomized controlled trial published in *Traumatology*, participants with PTSD who underwent EFT sessions showed significant reductions in both the severity of symptoms and overall emotional distress. Another study in the *Journal of Clinical Psychology* found that EFT was as effective, if not more so, than traditional talk therapy in reducing symptoms of anxiety, with improvements sustained even after follow-up assessments. These studies suggest that EFT can provide long-term emotional relief, particularly for those suffering from trauma-related conditions.

EFT has also been studied for its potential benefits in **pain management**. Research has shown that the technique can significantly reduce chronic pain, particularly when emotional components are involved. In a study published in *Integrative Medicine: A Clinician's Journal*, participants with chronic pain conditions, such as fibromyalgia and chronic fatigue syndrome, experienced substantial pain relief after EFT treatment. The reduction in pain was linked to both the emotional healing process and the direct impact of tapping on the body's energy system, which may help alleviate muscle tension and promote relaxation.

The **neurological effects** of EFT have also been explored through brain imaging and other advanced techniques. A study using functional magnetic resonance imaging (fMRI) found that EFT significantly reduced activity in the amygdala, the part of the brain associated with the processing of fear and anxiety. This reduction in amygdala activity suggests that EFT may help rewire the brain's response to stress and emotional triggers. Additionally, brainwave research using electroencephalography (EEG) has shown that EFT can shift brainwave patterns, moving individuals from a highly aroused state (characterized by beta waves) to a more relaxed and calm state (characterized by alpha and theta waves). These shifts in brain activity support the idea that EFT can induce a state of relaxation and emotional regulation.

In terms of **emotional regulation**, studies have found that EFT helps individuals better manage their emotions by increasing self-awareness and mindfulness. One study published in *Psychological Reports* showed that participants who underwent EFT therapy demonstrated significant improvements in emotional regulation, as well as reductions in negative emotions such as anger, fear, and sadness. The study concluded that EFT's focus on tapping while verbalizing distressing emotions helps individuals process and release emotional blockages, leading to enhanced emotional clarity and well-being.

Another area of interest in recent research is the **placebo effect** in EFT. While some may argue that the results are primarily driven by belief or expectation, studies have shown that the benefits of EFT go beyond placebo. A study published in *Energy Psychology: Theory, Research & Treatment* demonstrated that EFT produced substantial improvements in anxiety and depression, which were not only evident immediately after treatment but were also sustained at follow-up sessions. The researchers concluded that the results were not merely the result of placebo, as the improvements were measurable and beyond what would be expected from suggestive or placebo treatments alone.

In the context of **weight loss and cravings**, EFT has shown promise as well. A study published in *The Journal of Nutrition and Metabolism* explored the effects of EFT on individuals with food cravings. The study found that participants who used EFT to address emotional triggers around eating experienced significant reductions in cravings and improved dietary choices. These findings suggest that EFT could be an effective tool for addressing emotional eating and fostering healthier lifestyle habits.

The growing body of evidence on EFT also underscores its **versatility** as a therapeutic tool. From improving emotional resilience to providing relief from physical pain, EFT has been shown to benefit a wide range of individuals, regardless of their specific issues. The technique's holistic approach—addressing both the emotional and physical components of distress—makes it a unique and effective option for managing stress, trauma, pain, and other health concerns.

As more studies are conducted, the scientific community continues to explore the mechanisms behind EFT's effectiveness. While much of the research is still in its early stages, the results thus far have been promising, indicating that EFT is a valuable tool in both clinical and self-help contexts. As the research base grows, EFT is likely to gain even wider acceptance as a legitimate and scientifically supported therapeutic technique for emotional and physical healing.

EFT and Stress Management

Stress is a natural response to life's challenges, but when it becomes chronic, it can negatively affect both emotional and physical health. Research has shown that ongoing stress is linked to a variety of conditions, including anxiety, depression, cardiovascular issues, and even chronic pain. Emotional Freedom Technique (EFT) has emerged as a powerful tool for managing stress by addressing both the psychological and physiological aspects of stress.

One of the key ways in which EFT works for stress management is through its ability to reduce the body's **stress response**. When the brain perceives a threat, it triggers the "fight or flight" response, activating the sympathetic nervous system. This results in the release of stress hormones, such as cortisol and adrenaline, which prepare the body to respond to the danger. While this response is essential in acute situations, chronic activation of this system can be detrimental, leading to health problems like high blood pressure, weakened immune function, and emotional burnout. EFT aims to calm this stress response by stimulating specific acupressure points, which activates the parasympathetic nervous system—the body's "rest and digest" mode—thereby reducing the effects of stress.

Cortisol levels are a key physiological marker of stress, and EFT has been shown to significantly lower cortisol levels. Studies have demonstrated that a single EFT session can result in a noticeable reduction in cortisol, sometimes by as much as 40% to 50%. This immediate reduction in cortisol not only helps the body return to a balanced state but also supports emotional regulation, as high cortisol levels are often associated with feelings of anxiety, tension, and irritability. By reducing cortisol, EFT helps individuals feel more relaxed and centered, allowing them to better cope with stressful situations.

EFT also provides an **effective tool for emotional regulation**, a critical component in stress management. Chronic stress often results in emotional dysregulation, where individuals feel overwhelmed by their emotions, making it difficult to manage day-to-day challenges. EFT helps individuals process and release pent-up emotions by focusing on the emotional trigger while tapping on acupressure points. This combination of physical and psychological interventions creates a sense of emotional balance, helping individuals respond to stressors in a more measured, calm way.

One of the primary benefits of EFT in stress management is its **self-regulation capability**. Unlike many therapeutic techniques, which require a trained professional,

EFT can be practiced on one's own, giving individuals the tools to manage stress in real-time. Whether in the middle of a stressful workday or when facing a personal challenge, EFT can be used to reduce stress and regain composure. This sense of autonomy is empowering, as it enables individuals to take control of their emotional well-being, without relying solely on external resources or medication.

The **relaxation effect** of EFT is often immediate. As individuals tap on the meridian points while focusing on the issue at hand, they often report feeling a sense of calm and relaxation almost immediately. This relaxation effect is linked to changes in brain activity. Functional MRI studies have shown that EFT can reduce activity in the amygdala, the brain's emotional center that processes fear and anxiety, while increasing activity in the prefrontal cortex, which is responsible for decision-making and emotional regulation. This shift in brain activity helps individuals process stressful emotions with greater clarity and less reactivity, making it easier to navigate stressful situations.

In addition to its direct impact on stress hormones and brain activity, EFT also helps to address the **root causes of stress**. For many individuals, stress arises not just from external pressures but also from internal beliefs, fears, and unresolved emotional issues. EFT allows individuals to focus on these underlying emotional triggers, such as past trauma, anxiety, or negative self-talk, and neutralize them. This helps to break the cycle of stress by targeting not just the immediate symptoms but also the deeper emotional patterns that contribute to long-term stress. As these emotional blockages are released, individuals may feel a greater sense of peace and a reduced emotional burden.

Long-term stress can also contribute to physical tension, especially in areas like the neck, shoulders, and back. Chronic stress can cause muscle tightness, which, over time, can result in chronic pain and discomfort. EFT has been shown to help alleviate this muscle tension by addressing both the emotional and physical components of stress. As emotional distress is released, the body's muscle tension often dissipates, leading to a feeling of physical relaxation and relief.

EFT's ability to improve **sleep quality** also plays a role in stress management. Sleep disturbances are common in individuals experiencing chronic stress, anxiety, or depression. By reducing the physical and emotional markers of stress, EFT helps individuals achieve a state of relaxation conducive to better sleep. Studies have shown that individuals who use EFT to address their stress report improved sleep quality, falling asleep more easily and experiencing fewer awakenings during the night. This restorative sleep is essential for recovery and overall well-being.

The scientific evidence supporting EFT for stress management is also growing. In addition to cortisol reduction, studies have shown that EFT can improve measures of **heart rate variability (HRV)**, which is a marker of the body's ability to adapt to stress. Higher HRV is associated with better emotional resilience and overall health, while low

HRV is a sign of chronic stress and poor health. EFT has been found to increase HRV, further confirming its effectiveness in reducing stress and improving overall physiological functioning.

In conclusion, EFT offers a holistic and effective approach to stress management, addressing both the physiological and psychological aspects of stress. By reducing cortisol levels, calming the nervous system, improving emotional regulation, and addressing the root causes of stress, EFT provides individuals with a powerful tool to manage stress in a healthy and sustainable way. Whether used as a daily practice or in response to specific stressors, EFT can help individuals navigate the challenges of life with greater ease, resilience, and emotional balance.

How EFT can manage stress

EFT offers a unique and effective way to manage stress by combining elements of cognitive therapy with acupressure. Stress is often a result of both emotional and physical factors, and EFT targets both of these aspects, providing a comprehensive approach to stress management.

At the core of EFT's effectiveness in managing stress is its ability to **regulate the body's stress response**. When we encounter a stressful situation, our body enters a heightened state of alertness, activating the "fight or flight" response. This triggers the release of stress hormones like cortisol and adrenaline, which prepare the body to deal with the perceived threat. While this response is essential for short-term challenges, prolonged activation of the stress response can lead to negative health outcomes, including anxiety, high blood pressure, and chronic fatigue. EFT helps to **calm the body's nervous system** by tapping on specific acupressure points while focusing on the emotional issue at hand. This tapping is thought to stimulate the body's energy system, restoring balance and reducing the intensity of the stress response.

One of the most significant ways EFT helps manage stress is by **lowering cortisol levels**. Cortisol, the primary stress hormone, is produced by the adrenal glands in response to stress. High levels of cortisol, when sustained over time, can lead to anxiety, depression, and physical ailments. Research has shown that EFT can significantly reduce cortisol levels, with some studies reporting up to a 40% reduction in cortisol after a single tapping session. By lowering cortisol, EFT helps the body return to a more relaxed state, reducing both the emotional and physical symptoms of stress.

EFT also aids in **emotional regulation**. Chronic stress often leads to emotional dysregulation, where individuals feel overwhelmed, anxious, or unable to cope with daily challenges. The process of tapping while focusing on specific emotional triggers helps individuals bring awareness to the underlying emotional issues causing stress. By acknowledging these emotions and tapping on the acupressure points, the emotional intensity is thought to decrease, leading to a more balanced emotional state. This helps individuals respond to stressors with greater calmness and clarity, rather than reacting impulsively or feeling overwhelmed.

Another benefit of EFT is its ability to **shift the brain's response to stress**. Studies using brain imaging techniques, such as functional MRI, have shown that EFT reduces activity in the amygdala, the brain's fear center. The amygdala is responsible for processing emotions like fear and anxiety, and when it is overactive, it can amplify the stress response. By calming the amygdala, EFT helps the brain process stress in a more regulated way, making it easier to handle emotional triggers without becoming overwhelmed. Additionally, EFT has been shown to increase activity in the prefrontal cortex, the area of the brain responsible for decision-making, emotional regulation, and rational thought. This shift in brain activity helps individuals approach stressors with a clearer, more logical perspective.

EFT also addresses the **physical manifestations of stress**. Chronic stress can lead to muscle tension, headaches, and other physical symptoms, which only exacerbate feelings of anxiety and discomfort. By tapping on specific acupressure points, EFT promotes the relaxation of muscles and alleviates physical tension. This helps to counteract the physical effects of stress, such as tightness in the neck, shoulders, and back, providing relief and promoting a sense of calm.

One of the unique aspects of EFT is its **self-administered nature**. Unlike many therapeutic techniques, which require a therapist or specialized setting, EFT can be practiced on your own, giving you the tools to manage stress at any time. Whether you're feeling anxious before a big presentation, overwhelmed by a personal issue, or simply stressed by the demands of daily life, EFT allows you to address the emotional and physical components of stress in real time. This accessibility makes EFT a highly practical and empowering stress management tool.

Additionally, **long-term stress** often stems from unresolved emotional issues or negative thought patterns, such as fear, guilt, or limiting beliefs. EFT helps address these underlying emotional causes by tapping on meridian points while focusing on the specific beliefs or experiences that are contributing to stress. By neutralizing these emotional blockages, EFT helps individuals release the emotional charge tied to these past experiences, reducing the impact they have on present-day stress levels.

EFT also promotes **mindfulness and self-awareness**, which are essential components of stress management. The technique encourages individuals to tune into their thoughts, feelings, and physical sensations, which fosters a greater understanding of the sources of stress and how they react to it. By becoming more aware of emotional triggers, individuals can learn to respond to stress more effectively, rather than reacting automatically or getting caught in a cycle of stress.

Finally, **EFT's ability to improve sleep** plays a crucial role in stress management. Chronic stress can interfere with sleep patterns, leading to insomnia or poor sleep quality. EFT helps by reducing stress and anxiety, calming the mind, and preparing the body for restful sleep. Improved sleep not only helps individuals recover from the physical effects of stress but also enhances emotional resilience, making it easier to cope with future stressors.

In conclusion, EFT is an effective, holistic tool for managing stress by addressing both the emotional and physical components of stress. By reducing cortisol levels, regulating the nervous system, improving emotional regulation, and promoting physical relaxation, EFT helps individuals cope with the demands of daily life with greater ease and resilience. Whether used as a preventative tool for stress or as an immediate solution to specific stressors, EFT empowers individuals to take control of their emotional well-being and achieve a greater sense of balance and calm.

Stress relief is essential for maintaining both emotional and physical well-being. Emotional Freedom Technique (EFT) offers a unique and effective approach to alleviating stress by combining tapping on acupressure points with focused attention on the emotional or physical issue at hand. This powerful combination can help to reset the body's stress response and promote a state of relaxation.

One of the core **EFT techniques** for stress relief is the **basic tapping sequence**. This involves tapping on a series of acupressure points located on the head, face, and upper body while focusing on a specific stressful situation or feeling. The points include the top of the head, the eyebrow, the side of the eye, under the eye, under the nose, the chin, the collarbone, and under the arm. By tapping on these points, you are stimulating the body's energy pathways, which can help release emotional blockages and promote relaxation. The process is simple, effective, and can be done anywhere, making it an ideal tool for managing stress in real time.

When using EFT for stress relief, the first step is to **identify the stressor**. This could be an emotional issue, such as anxiety about a work presentation, or a physical stressor, like tension in the neck and shoulders. Once the stressor is identified, rate the intensity of the stress on a scale from 0 to 10, with 10 being the highest level of distress. This helps to gauge the effectiveness of the session and track progress. Next, you create a **setup statement** that acknowledges the stress while also affirming self-acceptance. For example, "Even though I feel stressed about this presentation, I deeply and completely accept myself." This statement helps to address the emotional aspect of stress and sets a positive tone for the tapping process.

After the setup statement, you begin the **tapping sequence**, focusing on the specific stressor at each acupressure point. While tapping, it is important to stay connected to the emotions or physical sensations related to the stress, allowing the mind and body to process and release these feelings. This allows the body's energy system to reset, reducing the intensity of the stress response. Throughout the tapping process, you may notice a decrease in emotional charge and physical tension, signaling that the stress is being addressed at both the cognitive and energetic levels.

Another effective technique for **stress relief** with EFT is the use of **affirmations**. While tapping on the acupressure points, you can repeat positive affirmations that counteract negative thought patterns associated with stress. For example, if you're feeling overwhelmed, you might say, "I am calm and capable," or "I trust that I can handle this situation." These affirmations work in tandem with the tapping to shift your mindset and create a sense of empowerment and control, helping to release negative emotions and create a more balanced emotional state.

For deeper stress relief, EFT can be paired with **deep breathing exercises**. Stress often causes shallow, rapid breathing, which activates the body's stress response. By incorporating slow, deep breaths into your tapping routine, you can enhance the relaxation effect. As you tap, take long, deep breaths—inhale for a count of four, hold for a count of four, and exhale for a count of four. This breathing pattern calms the nervous system, reducing the physiological effects of stress while also allowing you to stay focused on the emotional aspects during the tapping process.

Visualizations can also be a powerful tool in EFT for stress relief. During the tapping session, you can imagine yourself in a peaceful place or visualize the stressful situation dissipating. For example, if you're feeling stressed about an upcoming meeting, you might visualize yourself walking into the room confidently, feeling calm and in control. This mental imagery, combined with tapping, can help reduce anxiety and increase feelings of self-assurance.

EFT for stress relief can also be used to address physical symptoms of stress, such as muscle tension or headaches. If you're experiencing tension in a specific area, you can focus on that part of the body during the tapping session. For example, if you have tight shoulders, you can tap while visualizing the tension melting away, or use specific language such as, "Even though I have this tightness in my shoulders, I choose to relax and release it." This helps to target the physical manifestation of stress, promoting a sense of relaxation and comfort.

In addition to the basic tapping techniques, **advanced EFT techniques** can be used for deeper emotional release. One such method is **the tearless trauma technique**, which involves tapping on acupressure points while focusing on a stressful or traumatic memory, but without verbalizing the details of the event. This method can be particularly useful for those who find it difficult to talk about their stressors or trauma. By focusing on the physical sensations of stress without re-living the emotional pain, this technique helps to process and release the stored tension and emotional charge.

Another advanced technique is the **chasing the pain method**, which involves following the sensations of discomfort or tension in the body. This approach can be particularly helpful for individuals who experience chronic stress-related pain, such as headaches, back pain, or digestive issues. By tapping on specific points while focusing on the location of pain, the body's energy system can begin to release the blockages that contribute to the physical discomfort.

For those who experience **ongoing stress or anxiety**, using EFT as a regular practice can help to build emotional resilience and reduce overall stress levels. Consistent tapping sessions allow individuals to process daily stressors in a healthy, proactive way, preventing emotional build-up and offering long-term stress relief. By incorporating EFT into your routine, you can create a powerful habit of self-care, strengthening your ability to cope with stress in a calm and balanced manner.

In conclusion, EFT provides a diverse array of techniques for relieving stress, from basic tapping sequences to advanced methods designed for deeper emotional and physical release. By targeting both the emotional and physical aspects of stress, EFT offers a holistic approach that can help restore balance, promote relaxation, and increase emotional resilience. Whether used in response to a specific stressor or as part of an ongoing self-care routine, EFT empowers individuals to take control of their stress and cultivate a greater sense of well-being.

Case studies of stress management with EFT

Numerous case studies have demonstrated the effectiveness of Emotional Freedom Technique (EFT) in managing stress across various settings, from corporate environments to therapeutic contexts. These case studies provide valuable insights into how EFT can reduce stress, promote emotional well-being, and support individuals in regaining control over their emotional responses.

Case Study 1: Workplace Stress Reduction A 2016 study published in the *Journal of Nervous and Mental Disease* explored the effects of EFT on workplace stress. The study involved 50 employees from a high-pressure corporate setting, many of whom reported high levels of work-related stress, anxiety, and burnout. Over the course of four EFT sessions, participants learned the basic tapping sequence and were encouraged to use EFT during particularly stressful moments. The results were remarkable: at the end of the study, 80% of participants reported a significant reduction in stress levels, with a decrease in self-reported anxiety and a noticeable improvement in overall mood. Furthermore, the study participants showed a reduction in **cortisol levels**, the body's primary stress hormone, which was measured before and after each session. This study highlighted EFT's ability to not only reduce the emotional experience of stress but also its biological markers, such as cortisol, supporting the technique's effectiveness in managing workplace stress.

Case Study 2: EFT for Chronic Anxiety and Stress Relief A clinical case study published in the *International Journal of Stress Management* focused on a 35-year-old woman who had struggled with chronic anxiety and stress for over a decade. She had a history of panic attacks, high anxiety levels, and insomnia, all of which were exacerbated by a demanding job and personal issues. Traditional therapy and medication had provided limited relief. After undergoing 8 weeks of EFT treatment, the woman reported dramatic improvements. Her anxiety decreased significantly, and she was able to manage work-related stress more effectively. Additionally, her sleep quality improved, and she was able to focus more on her work without being overwhelmed by the constant pressure. One key outcome of this case study was the marked reduction in her **physical symptoms of anxiety**, including muscle tension, headaches, and gastrointestinal issues, which she had associated with stress for years. EFT's ability to address both the emotional and physical symptoms of stress played a pivotal role in her recovery.

Case Study 3: Post-Traumatic Stress Disorder (PTSD) and Stress Relief In a case study of a combat veteran with PTSD, EFT was utilized as part of a broader treatment plan for stress and trauma. The veteran, a 42-year-old male, had experienced severe stress and emotional instability following his deployment in a war zone. He struggled with flashbacks, hypervigilance, irritability, and emotional numbness, symptoms consistent with PTSD. After 12 EFT sessions, his symptoms improved significantly, particularly in relation to the emotional triggers that had once set off intense stress responses. He reported feeling more emotionally balanced, with a reduction in flashbacks and a decrease in the frequency of panic attacks. In addition to the emotional benefits, the veteran also experienced a **reduction in physical tension**—he described his muscles feeling "less tight" and his overall body feeling more relaxed. This case study is a testament to how EFT can help individuals with deep emotional wounds process and manage stress, providing long-term relief.

Case Study 4: School Teacher's Stress Management A 29-year-old school teacher participated in a case study exploring EFT as a means of managing stress in an educational environment. Teaching can be an incredibly stressful profession, and the participant struggled with feelings of overwhelm, burnout, and the pressure of meeting the expectations of both students and administration. After learning and applying EFT in five sessions, she noticed a significant reduction in stress levels. She found that tapping helped her process the frustrations and anxieties that accumulated throughout the day, allowing her to feel calmer and more present with her students. Her reported **work-related stress scores** decreased by over 50%, and she felt more confident in her ability to handle challenging classroom situations. This case study underscores the versatility of EFT as a tool for stress management, especially in high-pressure professions.

Case Study 5: EFT for Student Stress and Anxiety A group of 30 high school students participated in a research study exploring the use of EFT to manage academic stress. The students, all of whom reported high levels of test anxiety and stress related to academic performance, were taught the EFT tapping sequence and asked to use it before studying or taking exams. Over the course of a semester, the students reported feeling more relaxed during tests and found that their overall stress levels had decreased. Teachers observed an improvement in **academic performance**, particularly in students who had previously experienced anxiety-related difficulties. In follow-up surveys, 75% of the students reported feeling more in control of their stress and better equipped to handle academic pressures. This case study suggests that EFT is an effective tool for young people dealing with the pressures of school and academic achievement.

Case Study 6: Chronic Pain and Stress Relief A patient with chronic pain, resulting from long-term stress and emotional trauma, participated in a case study to assess the impact of EFT on both pain levels and emotional well-being. The individual, a 50-year-old woman, had been experiencing persistent pain in her back and shoulders, which had worsened over the years. During the EFT sessions, she focused on both the emotional stress and the physical sensations of pain. Over the course of several weeks, she reported significant **pain reduction**, describing her symptoms as less intense and more manageable. Additionally, her emotional state improved as the emotional stress related to her pain was processed. This case study emphasizes EFT's potential to address the **mind-body connection**, as the release of emotional blockages can result in tangible physical relief.

In conclusion, these case studies highlight the versatility and effectiveness of EFT in managing stress. From workplace stress to PTSD, academic pressure, and chronic pain, EFT has proven to be a valuable tool for reducing emotional distress and enhancing overall well-being. The combination of acupressure and cognitive focus in EFT appears to address both the physiological and psychological components of stress, providing individuals with a holistic approach to managing their emotions and improving their quality of life. These real-world applications underscore EFT's potential as a therapeutic intervention for stress relief, offering hope and healing for those seeking natural, accessible solutions to emotional and physical stress.

EFT and Anxiety Disorders

Anxiety disorders are among the most common mental health issues, affecting millions of people worldwide. These disorders can range from generalized anxiety and panic attacks to social anxiety and specific phobias, each marked by persistent worry, fear, and unease. While traditional therapies like cognitive-behavioral therapy (CBT) and medication are often effective, many individuals are seeking additional or alternative approaches to manage their anxiety. One such approach that has gained significant attention is Emotional Freedom Technique (EFT), a powerful tool that combines acupressure and psychological techniques to reduce anxiety symptoms and promote emotional well-being.

EFT works by tapping on specific acupressure points on the body while focusing on the anxious thoughts, emotions, or physical sensations that are causing distress. These points are part of the body's energy system, and the tapping is believed to help release blockages in the energy flow that can contribute to emotional and physical tension. By stimulating these acupressure points, EFT can help reset the body's stress response, lower cortisol levels, and reduce the intensity of anxiety. This makes EFT a compelling option for people with anxiety disorders, offering a holistic and non-invasive approach to managing anxiety.

How EFT Works for Anxiety

The process of using EFT for anxiety involves two main components: the **psychological focus** and the **physical tapping**. The individual first identifies the source of their anxiety—whether it's a specific event, ongoing worry, or generalized feelings of unease. While focusing on the issue, the person taps on various acupressure points along the body's energy meridians. These points include areas on the head, face, and upper body, which correspond to key energy pathways. The combination of focusing on the emotional distress and tapping on the acupressure points is believed to send signals to the brain and the body, helping to regulate the stress response.

One of the central theories behind EFT's effectiveness is its ability to balance the body's **energy system**, which is thought to be disrupted during times of emotional distress, including anxiety. Traditional Chinese medicine posits that the flow of energy, or "qi," in the body is vital for physical and emotional health. When this flow is blocked or unbalanced, emotional problems like anxiety can arise. By tapping on the acupressure points, EFT is believed to restore balance, allowing the body's energy to flow freely, which can alleviate the physical symptoms of anxiety, such as tension, rapid heart rate, and shallow breathing.

EFT also helps with **cognitive reframing**. When tapping, individuals focus on the negative thoughts or beliefs fueling their anxiety. For example, someone with social anxiety might think, "I'm going to embarrass myself at the party." During an EFT session, they would tap while repeating a setup statement like, "Even though I have this fear of embarrassing myself, I deeply and completely accept myself." This process allows individuals to confront their anxious thoughts in a non-judgmental way while also sending signals to the brain that help reduce the emotional charge associated with those thoughts. Over time, this helps change the way the brain responds to anxiety-provoking situations, making them less overwhelming and more manageable.

Scientific Evidence Supporting EFT for Anxiety

Scientific studies have begun to validate EFT's effectiveness in treating anxiety disorders. One prominent study published in *Energy Psychology: Theory, Research & Treatment* demonstrated that EFT was effective in reducing symptoms of generalized anxiety disorder (GAD). In this study, participants who received just a few sessions of EFT experienced significant reductions in anxiety levels compared to those who received no treatment or were treated with other techniques. Another study published in the *Journal of Nervous and Mental Disease* found that EFT led to a substantial decrease in **cortisol levels,** the body's primary stress hormone, which plays a central role in the anxiety response. The reduction in cortisol levels supports the idea that EFT is effective in calming the body's stress response, a key element in managing anxiety.

Additional research has shown that EFT can be particularly effective for people suffering from **panic attacks**. Panic attacks are intense bursts of fear and physical symptoms, such as rapid heart rate, dizziness, and shortness of breath. In a clinical trial involving individuals with panic disorder, participants who received EFT treatment reported fewer panic attacks and a reduction in the severity of their anxiety symptoms. EFT's ability to regulate the autonomic nervous system, which controls the body's stress response, is believed to play a critical role in alleviating these symptoms.

EFT for Specific Anxiety Disorders

EFT has also been shown to be effective for a variety of specific anxiety disorders. For example, individuals with **social anxiety** have reported significant improvements after using EFT. Social anxiety is characterized by a fear of being judged or embarrassed in social situations. By using EFT, individuals can tap on the thoughts and physical sensations associated with social anxiety, such as the fear of being judged, the nervousness before public speaking, or the discomfort in large groups. EFT helps release the emotional charge around these fears and replaces negative beliefs with more empowering ones, such as "I am confident in social situations" or "I am comfortable speaking in front of others." This cognitive shift can lead to more relaxed social interactions and less avoidance of social settings.

EFT for Test Anxiety

Students who experience **test anxiety** often feel overwhelmed and incapacitated by the fear of failing. This anxiety can interfere with their ability to study, concentrate, or perform during exams. EFT has been used effectively to help students reduce test-related stress by tapping on the emotions and thoughts that arise before or during exams. In a study involving students with test anxiety, participants who practiced EFT before exams experienced improved performance, reduced anxiety, and greater confidence. EFT's ability to regulate emotional responses to pressure and improve focus makes it a valuable tool for managing test anxiety.

EFT for Generalized Anxiety Disorder (GAD)

Generalized Anxiety Disorder (GAD) involves excessive and uncontrollable worry about everyday events. Individuals with GAD may experience chronic anxiety over matters like work, relationships, or health, often without a specific trigger. EFT has shown promise in alleviating the symptoms of GAD by helping individuals confront the root causes of their anxiety. By tapping while focusing on the worries and fears associated with GAD, individuals can process and release these emotions, helping to reduce the overall anxiety levels. One study found that individuals with GAD who used EFT experienced significant reductions in anxiety, depression, and physical symptoms after just a few sessions of tapping.

EFT is a promising and effective tool for managing anxiety disorders, providing a holistic approach that addresses both the emotional and physical aspects of anxiety. By tapping on specific acupressure points and focusing on the thoughts and emotions tied to anxiety, EFT can help individuals release the emotional charge of anxiety-provoking situations, reduce physical symptoms, and promote a greater sense of calm. With growing scientific evidence supporting its efficacy, EFT is becoming an increasingly popular option for those seeking a natural, accessible, and non-invasive way to manage anxiety and improve their emotional well-being. Whether used alongside other therapeutic interventions or as a standalone approach, EFT offers a powerful tool for individuals dealing with anxiety in its many forms.

Application of EFT to anxiety

Anxiety, whether it manifests as persistent worry, panic attacks, or generalized unease, can significantly impact daily life. Many people seek ways to alleviate these feelings, and one such method gaining attention is **Emotional Freedom Technique (EFT)**. EFT offers a unique, non-invasive approach to managing anxiety by combining tapping on acupressure points with focused attention on emotional distress. This technique has proven effective in addressing both the emotional and physical components of anxiety, helping individuals regain control and reduce the overwhelming feelings often associated with the disorder.

How EFT Targets Anxiety

EFT works by tapping on specific acupressure points, which are thought to correspond to energy pathways or meridians in the body. According to traditional Chinese medicine, blockages or disruptions in the body's energy flow can lead to emotional issues such as anxiety. By tapping on these points while focusing on the specific anxiety-provoking thought, memory, or feeling, EFT helps to clear the emotional blocks and restore balance to the body's energy system. This process is thought to recalibrate the nervous system, calming the body's natural fight-or-flight response and helping the individual regain a sense of emotional balance.

The process begins with identifying the **specific source of anxiety**, whether it's a particular situation, general worry, or a specific phobia. While focusing on this anxiety trigger, the individual taps on a sequence of acupressure points, such as the top of the head, eyebrows, sides of the eyes, under the eyes, under the nose, chin, collarbone, and under the arms. This tapping helps reduce the intensity of the anxiety by signaling to the brain that the body is safe, thus lowering the stress response. The goal is to **reduce the emotional charge** connected to the anxious thought or event, making it less distressing over time.

EFT and Emotional Recalibration

The emotional aspect of anxiety often includes intrusive thoughts, worries about the future, or intense fears of what could go wrong. These thoughts can lead to a cascade of physical symptoms such as rapid heart rate, shallow breathing, sweating, and muscle tension. EFT addresses both components: the emotional and physical. As the individual taps on the acupressure points, they not only focus on their anxious thoughts but also on the **physical sensations** associated with those emotions, such as the tightness in their chest or the butterflies in their stomach. By tapping on these points, EFT helps to **release** these uncomfortable sensations, leading to a greater sense of relaxation and emotional clarity.

Steps for Using EFT to Manage Anxiety

The process of using EFT to manage anxiety typically involves several key steps:

1. **Identify the Source of Anxiety**: Begin by pinpointing the exact cause of anxiety—whether it's a specific event, general life stressors, or a long-standing fear or worry.
2. **Rate the Intensity**: On a scale from 0 to 10, rate how intense the anxiety feels. This helps measure progress during the session and gauge how effective the tapping is in reducing the anxiety.
3. **Create a Setup Statement**: A key part of EFT involves acknowledging the anxiety while also practicing **self-acceptance**. A common setup statement might be: "Even though I feel anxious about this meeting, I deeply and completely accept myself." This helps address any negative self-talk and promotes self-compassion during the process.
4. **Begin Tapping**: Start tapping on the designated acupressure points while repeating a reminder phrase, such as, "This anxiety," or, "This fear about the meeting." The goal is to stay focused on the anxiety while tapping, which helps release the emotional charge tied to the event or thought.
5. **Re-evaluate**: After completing a round of tapping, re-rate the intensity of the anxiety on the 0-10 scale. If the anxiety has decreased, you can repeat the tapping with a new statement or continue tapping on other aspects of the anxiety. If the intensity remains high, continue tapping until there's a noticeable reduction in emotional distress.

Specific Applications of EFT for Anxiety

EFT can be tailored to address various forms of anxiety, including:

1. **Generalized Anxiety Disorder (GAD)**: For individuals who experience chronic, excessive worry about everyday situations, EFT can help break the cycle of worry. By focusing on the specific worries and tapping on them, EFT helps individuals develop a sense of **control** over their anxiety, making it more manageable and less overwhelming.
2. **Social Anxiety**: Many people struggle with the fear of being judged or making mistakes in social situations. EFT can help individuals tap on the specific fears they experience in social settings, such as the fear of public speaking, talking to strangers, or even being in large groups. Over time, tapping helps reduce the

emotional intensity of these fears, making social situations feel more **comfortable** and less intimidating.

3. **Panic Attacks**: Panic attacks are characterized by intense feelings of fear and physical symptoms such as heart palpitations, dizziness, and shortness of breath. EFT can be used both to prevent and manage panic attacks by addressing the **fear of future attacks** as well as the physical sensations during an episode. Tapping on the points associated with the chest, heart, and head can help regulate the body's stress response, reducing the likelihood or severity of a panic attack.
4. **Phobias**: Specific phobias, such as a fear of flying or heights, often result in intense anxiety when exposed to the trigger. EFT works by focusing on the fear while tapping, gradually desensitizing the individual to the object of their fear. This process allows the emotional charge to dissipate over time, making the phobia less overpowering.
5. **Performance Anxiety**: For those who experience anxiety before exams, presentations, or performances, EFT can be a highly effective tool for reducing **nervousness** and enhancing performance. Tapping before or during an event helps calm the nerves and shift focus away from fear of failure, allowing individuals to feel more **confident** and prepared.

Scientific Backing for EFT and Anxiety

Numerous studies have shown the effectiveness of EFT for reducing anxiety. Research published in the *Journal of Nervous and Mental Disease* has demonstrated that EFT not only reduces the **symptoms of anxiety** but also lowers cortisol levels, which are associated with the body's stress response. Another study published in *Energy Psychology: Theory, Research & Treatment* found that individuals who used EFT reported a significant decrease in anxiety and associated symptoms after just a few sessions. These findings highlight the potential of EFT as a powerful tool in managing anxiety disorders, offering a natural and accessible solution for those looking to reduce stress and regain emotional balance.

EFT as a Complementary Tool

While EFT is highly effective on its own, it can also be used alongside other therapies, such as cognitive-behavioral therapy (CBT), medication, or mindfulness practices. In fact, many people find that EFT helps them process emotions and reinforce the strategies they learn in traditional therapy. Its ability to work with both the **mind and body** makes it a comprehensive tool for managing anxiety and enhancing emotional well-being.

EFT offers an innovative, accessible, and effective method for addressing anxiety. By combining acupressure tapping with mental focus, EFT helps individuals process their anxiety, reduce physical symptoms, and shift their emotional response to stress. Whether used for generalized anxiety, panic attacks, social anxiety, or phobias, EFT offers a holistic approach to managing anxiety that works with the body's natural energy system to promote relaxation and emotional balance. With growing scientific support and numerous real-world success stories, EFT is increasingly recognized as a valuable tool for those seeking relief from anxiety in a natural and empowering way.

Simple techniques to cope with anxiety

When anxiety strikes, finding ways to manage the intense feelings of worry, fear, or nervousness can be crucial to regaining control. Emotional Freedom Technique (EFT) offers several simple, accessible techniques that can quickly alleviate anxiety and help restore a sense of calm. These techniques combine the power of acupressure tapping with focused attention on the emotional or physical symptoms of anxiety, providing immediate relief and helping to rewire the body's stress response.

1. The Basic EFT Tapping Sequence

One of the simplest ways to cope with anxiety using EFT is to perform the basic tapping sequence. This involves tapping on key acupressure points while focusing on the specific issue causing distress. Here's how to do it:

- **Identify the source of your anxiety**: This might be a specific event, a thought, or a physical sensation like tightness in the chest. Acknowledge the anxiety without judgment.
- **Rate the intensity**: On a scale of 0-10, rate how intense your anxiety feels. This helps track progress as you tap.
- **Create a setup statement**: This is a phrase that acknowledges your anxiety while practicing self-acceptance. For example: "Even though I feel anxious about this meeting, I deeply and completely accept myself."
- **Tap on the acupressure points**: Begin tapping gently on the following points while focusing on your anxiety:
    1. **Top of the Head** (Crown)
    2. **Eyebrow** (at the beginning of the brow, closest to the nose)
    3. **Side of the Eye** (on the bone near the outer corner of the eye)
    4. **Under the Eye** (on the bone below the eye)
    5. **Under the Nose** (between the nose and upper lip)
    6. **Chin** (in the crease of the chin)
    7. **Collarbone** (just below the collarbone, where the breastbone and collarbones meet)
    8. **Under the Arm** (about 4 inches below the armpit)
- **Repeat**: As you tap each point, repeat a reminder phrase, such as "This anxiety" or "I feel nervous about the presentation." Continue tapping until the intensity of your anxiety decreases.

- **Re-rate the intensity**: After a round of tapping, re-rate how strong your anxiety feels on the 0-10 scale. Repeat the tapping process as needed until the intensity reduces.

2. The "Surrender" Technique

If you're feeling overwhelmed by anxiety and don't know where to start, the "Surrender" technique can be incredibly helpful. This approach focuses on accepting the anxiety rather than trying to fight it.

- **Acknowledge the Anxiety**: Simply say, "I surrender to this anxiety," or "I allow myself to feel this anxiety."
- **Tap on the acupressure points** while you say this phrase or while focusing on the feeling of surrendering to the anxiety. As you tap, allow yourself to truly feel and accept the anxiety, without judgment or resistance.

This technique helps create a shift from fighting the anxiety to accepting it as it is, which can often reduce its intensity. In doing so, the body and mind move from a state of resistance (which only heightens anxiety) to a place of calm acceptance.

3. Breathing and Tapping Combination

For those who experience physical symptoms of anxiety, such as shallow breathing or a racing heart, combining tapping with deep breathing can be especially soothing. Here's a simple technique:

- **Take a deep breath**: Inhale deeply through your nose, allowing your stomach to expand. Hold the breath for a moment and then exhale slowly through your mouth.
- **Tap and breathe simultaneously**: While you are tapping on the acupressure points, continue to breathe deeply, focusing on calming your breath and body. The combination of tapping and controlled breathing helps activate the body's relaxation response, easing both the physical and emotional aspects of anxiety.
- **Continue for a few rounds**: Tap through the sequence while maintaining your deep, steady breathing. With each round, you may notice your heart rate slowing and your anxiety easing.

4. The "Even Though" Setup for Negative Emotions

If anxiety is tied to negative thoughts or self-criticism, the "Even Though" setup can be a powerful way to reframe those thoughts. The setup involves acknowledging the emotional distress while reassuring yourself with self-compassion.

- **Identify the underlying thought**: Anxiety often stems from negative thoughts like "I'm not prepared for this," or "What if I fail?"
- **Create an "Even Though" setup statement**: Acknowledge the fear while reassuring yourself. For example, "Even though I'm worried about failing the exam, I deeply and completely accept myself."
- **Tap on the acupressure points**: While tapping on each point, continue repeating the "Even Though" statement, gradually shifting to a more positive or neutral belief. For example, "Even though I feel anxious, I know I can handle this."

This technique helps reframe anxious thoughts, replacing self-criticism with self-compassion, which can reduce the anxiety and improve emotional resilience.

5. Quick Calming Tapping (Tapping for Panic)

For those who experience sudden panic attacks or extreme anxiety, a quick, targeted approach can be effective. This method uses a rapid tapping technique to calm the nervous system in a short amount of time:

- **Focus on the immediate feeling of panic**: Identify the sensations in your body, such as tightness in the chest, shortness of breath, or dizziness.
- **Tap rapidly on the top of the head** and **collarbone points**: These are two of the most powerful acupressure points for calming the body. Tap briskly on these points while focusing on your panic and consciously telling your body to relax.
- **Deep Breathing**: Continue to take deep breaths while tapping, allowing your body to reset and calm down. This process helps interrupt the physiological cycle of panic and stress.

By using this technique in moments of heightened anxiety, the body can quickly return to a more balanced state, reducing the physical and emotional intensity of the panic attack.

6. Tapping for Grounding

Anxiety often causes people to feel disconnected or out of control. A grounding technique can help restore a sense of safety and calm. To ground yourself, focus on the present moment while tapping through the points.

- **Focus on your feet**: Imagine you are connected to the ground beneath you, like roots growing into the earth. As you tap, imagine those roots growing deeper, helping you feel more centered and stable.
- **Use grounding phrases**: While tapping, repeat affirmations like "I am safe," "I am grounded," or "I am in control of this moment." The goal is to shift focus away from the anxiety and reconnect with a feeling of physical and emotional stability.

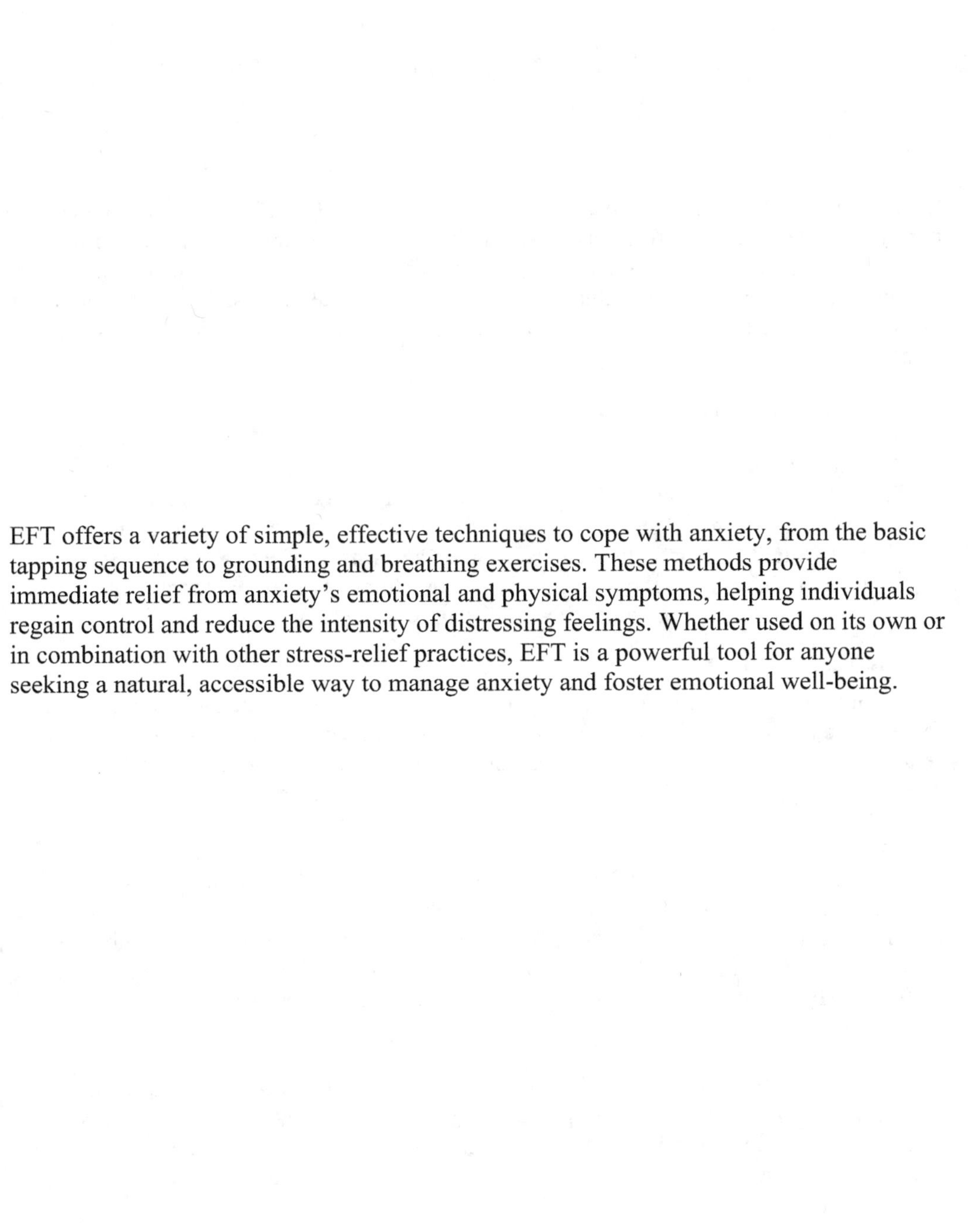

EFT offers a variety of simple, effective techniques to cope with anxiety, from the basic tapping sequence to grounding and breathing exercises. These methods provide immediate relief from anxiety's emotional and physical symptoms, helping individuals regain control and reduce the intensity of distressing feelings. Whether used on its own or in combination with other stress-relief practices, EFT is a powerful tool for anyone seeking a natural, accessible way to manage anxiety and foster emotional well-being.

Case studies and examples

Case studies and real-life examples of Emotional Freedom Technique (EFT) provide powerful evidence of its effectiveness in managing various emotional and psychological issues, including anxiety, stress, trauma, and phobias. These examples illustrate how EFT has been applied to real-world situations, offering a practical glimpse into its benefits and outcomes. Here are a few notable case studies that demonstrate the impact of this technique.

Case Study 1: Overcoming Generalized Anxiety Disorder (GAD)

Client Background:
Sarah, a 34-year-old woman, had been living with generalized anxiety disorder for over a decade. Her anxiety manifested in constant worry about work, relationships, and her health. She struggled with daily feelings of dread and was unable to relax, often experiencing tightness in her chest and shallow breathing. Traditional therapy had provided some relief, but her anxiety would return during periods of stress.

EFT Intervention:
After Sarah was introduced to EFT, she began tapping on the acupressure points while focusing on the thoughts and physical sensations associated with her anxiety. Her initial setup statement was, "Even though I feel anxious about everything in my life, I deeply and completely accept myself."

Outcome:
After just a few EFT sessions, Sarah reported a significant reduction in her anxiety levels. She was able to identify specific triggers and use tapping techniques to address them in the moment. With continued use of EFT, she learned to manage her anxiety without it overwhelming her daily life. Sarah's self-reported intensity of anxiety dropped from an 8/10 to a 2/10 on the anxiety scale after three weeks of consistent tapping.

:

This case highlights how EFT can be an effective tool for individuals dealing with generalized anxiety disorder. By targeting the emotional triggers and combining them with physical tapping, Sarah was able to regain a sense of control and calm, significantly reducing her anxiety levels.

Client Background:
James, a 45-year-old man, had been suffering from panic attacks for several years. His panic attacks were sudden and overwhelming, often triggered by stressful situations at work or social settings. The physical symptoms were intense: rapid heartbeat, shortness of breath, and a feeling of impending doom. James had tried medication and therapy, but nothing provided long-lasting relief.

EFT Intervention:
James was introduced to EFT as a way to address his panic attacks. During his first session, he tapped on the points while focusing on the feelings of anxiety and the physical sensations of panic. His setup statement was, "Even though I feel like I'm going to have a panic attack, I accept myself completely."

Outcome:
After a few tapping sessions, James learned how to apply EFT during the onset of a panic attack. By focusing on the anxiety and tapping through the sequence of points, James noticed that his physical symptoms began to subside much faster than they had in the past. He also reported that his overall anxiety levels decreased, and he was able to face stressors with greater resilience.

James was able to reduce the frequency and intensity of his panic attacks. Where he once experienced multiple panic attacks a week, he now had only one or two mild episodes per month.

:
This case shows how EFT can be a valuable tool for individuals suffering from panic attacks. Through tapping on the body's acupressure points and focusing on the physical and emotional symptoms of anxiety, individuals can regain control over their bodies and reduce the intensity of panic responses.

Client Background:
Laura, a 29-year-old woman, had a severe fear of flying that began when she experienced a turbulent flight during a trip abroad. This fear led to avoidance behavior, including refusing to travel for work or personal reasons. Laura had tried other therapies, but her fear persisted, limiting her opportunities for travel.

EFT Intervention:
Laura started working with an EFT practitioner who guided her through the process of tapping on her fear of flying. The practitioner asked her to recall the traumatic flight and

tap through the acupressure points while focusing on her fear. Her setup statement was, "Even though I feel terrified of flying, I choose to release this fear."

Outcome:
After a few sessions of tapping, Laura's emotional charge around flying was significantly reduced. She reported that when she thought about flying, her fear diminished from an 8/10 to a 2/10. With continued practice, Laura felt empowered to board a short flight, where she used EFT to manage her anxiety in real-time. By the end of the sessions, she was able to fly without experiencing the intense fear she once had.

:

This case demonstrates how EFT can be an effective tool for overcoming phobias, such as a fear of flying. By targeting the root emotional trauma and tapping through the acupressure points, EFT helped Laura break the cycle of fear and regain her ability to travel comfortably.

Case Study 4: Healing from Childhood Trauma

Client Background:
Mark, a 40-year-old man, had unresolved trauma from childhood abuse. He experienced feelings of shame, guilt, and anger related to his past, which affected his relationships and mental well-being. Despite years of therapy, he still struggled with emotional triggers related to the trauma.

EFT Intervention:
Mark began using EFT as part of a broader trauma-healing approach. He tapped on the acupressure points while focusing on specific memories of the abuse. His setup statement was, "Even though I carry this pain from my childhood, I choose to let it go."

Outcome:
After several sessions, Mark noticed a dramatic shift in how he viewed his past trauma. His emotional triggers—such as anger or shame—became less intense, and he could recall the events without becoming overwhelmed by negative emotions. Mark also reported feeling more at peace with himself and his past, which improved his relationships and sense of self-worth.

:

This case illustrates EFT's potential as a tool for healing deep emotional trauma. By tapping on traumatic memories while focusing on self-acceptance, Mark was able to release stored emotional energy and move toward emotional freedom.

Client Background:
Emily, a 38-year-old executive, was experiencing high levels of stress due to the demands of her job. She felt overwhelmed by deadlines, difficult clients, and the constant pressure to perform. This stress was affecting her health, sleep, and overall well-being.

EFT Intervention:
Emily learned EFT as a way to manage stress at work. She used the technique during stressful moments, tapping on the acupressure points while focusing on the anxiety related to her work. Her setup statement was, "Even though I feel so much pressure at work, I choose to relax and release this stress."

Outcome:
After incorporating EFT into her daily routine, Emily found that she could better manage stressful situations without letting them overwhelm her. She was able to regain perspective, improve her problem-solving abilities, and maintain a calmer state throughout the day. Over time, her physical symptoms of stress, such as tension in her shoulders and headaches, diminished.

:

EFT proved to be a valuable tool for managing workplace stress. By incorporating tapping into her daily routine, Emily was able to navigate the pressures of her high-demand job while maintaining her emotional and physical well-being.

These case studies illustrate the versatility and effectiveness of Emotional Freedom Technique (EFT) in managing a wide range of emotional and psychological challenges, including anxiety, panic attacks, phobias, trauma, and stress. The common thread across all these examples is the ability of EFT to address both the emotional and physical aspects of distress, providing individuals with a tool to manage their emotions and regain a sense of control. With continued practice and support, EFT has helped many individuals experience profound shifts in their emotional well-being, offering a path toward greater peace and emotional freedom.

EFT and Depression

Depression is a complex mental health condition that affects millions of people worldwide. It can manifest in a variety of ways, from persistent sadness and hopelessness to physical symptoms such as fatigue and changes in appetite. While traditional therapies, such as medication and talk therapy, have proven effective for many individuals, Emotional Freedom Technique (EFT) has emerged as a promising complementary treatment for managing and alleviating depression. By addressing both the emotional and physical components of the condition, EFT offers a holistic approach to healing.

How EFT Works for Depression

EFT is based on the concept that emotional distress and negative thought patterns can cause disruptions in the body's energy system, which is believed to influence physical and emotional health. The technique involves tapping on specific acupressure points on the body while focusing on negative emotions or traumatic memories. This combination of tapping and mental focus helps to clear emotional blockages and restore balance to the body's energy system, which is thought to help release negative emotions and alleviate symptoms of depression.

EFT and Negative Thought Patterns

One of the key mechanisms behind depression is the presence of persistent negative thought patterns. These thoughts often focus on feelings of worthlessness, guilt, or hopelessness, which can perpetuate the depressive cycle. EFT works by helping individuals confront these negative beliefs in a safe and non-judgmental manner. By tapping through the acupressure points while repeating phrases such as, "Even though I feel worthless, I deeply and completely accept myself," the individual is encouraged to reframe these thoughts and release the associated emotional charge.

Research suggests that EFT can help reduce the intensity of negative thought patterns by addressing the underlying emotional responses. By clearing the emotional blockages tied to these thoughts, EFT helps break the cycle of rumination that often keeps depression alive. The tapping process helps to "reset" the mind's response to negative thoughts, leading to a reduction in depressive symptoms over time.

EFT for Emotional and Physical Symptoms of Depression

Depression often manifests not only as a mental health issue but also as a physical one. Symptoms such as chronic fatigue, muscle tension, sleep disturbances, and changes in appetite are common in those who suffer from depression. EFT addresses both the emotional and physical symptoms simultaneously by working with the body's energy system.

For example, when someone is feeling depressed, they may experience a heavy feeling in their chest, a tightness in the throat, or a general sense of exhaustion. By tapping on acupressure points while focusing on these physical sensations, EFT can help release the energy blockages contributing to these symptoms. The physical tapping sends signals to the brain, promoting relaxation and reducing tension in the body, which can lead to improvements in mood, energy levels, and overall well-being.

Case Studies and Evidence for EFT's Effectiveness

Numerous studies and case reports have demonstrated the effectiveness of EFT in reducing depression symptoms. One study published in the *Journal of Nervous and Mental Disease* found that participants who received EFT treatments showed significant reductions in depression and anxiety levels. The study also found that EFT was more effective than traditional talk therapy in some cases, especially for individuals who had not responded well to other forms of treatment.

Another case study involved a woman named Jane, who had struggled with depression for over 15 years. Despite receiving traditional therapy and antidepressant medication, Jane's symptoms persisted, leaving her feeling hopeless. After several sessions of EFT, focusing on past trauma and self-worth issues, Jane reported a dramatic improvement in her mood. Her feelings of hopelessness and sadness decreased significantly, and she was able to regain her sense of joy and purpose. Jane's experience reflects the potential of EFT to provide lasting relief for those struggling with depression.

The Role of EFT in Trauma and Depression

Trauma is often closely linked with depression, particularly in cases where the individual has experienced significant emotional or physical abuse, loss, or betrayal. EFT has been shown to be highly effective in addressing trauma-related depression. By helping individuals process and release the emotional charge connected to traumatic events, EFT can provide a sense of relief and emotional release.

For example, a client dealing with childhood trauma might tap while focusing on a painful memory or feeling of abandonment. As they tap through the points, the emotional intensity of the memory decreases, allowing them to view the experience with less emotional reactivity. This release can help reduce the depressive symptoms that often accompany trauma, such as isolation, hopelessness, and sadness.

EFT as Part of a Holistic Approach to Depression

While EFT can be a powerful tool for alleviating depression, it is often most effective when used as part of a holistic treatment plan. Many people find that combining EFT with other therapeutic approaches—such as cognitive behavioral therapy (CBT), mindfulness practices, or physical exercise—can enhance the overall benefits.

EFT can also serve as a self-help tool that individuals can use at home. Once they have learned the technique, they can tap on their own to manage depressive symptoms as they arise. This makes EFT an empowering approach, as it provides individuals with a sense of control over their mental and emotional health.

Tips for Using EFT to Manage Depression

- **Focus on Specific Feelings**: When using EFT for depression, it is helpful to identify specific emotions or situations that are contributing to the depressive feelings. Focus on these feelings during tapping, using setup statements such as, "Even though I feel sad about my past, I choose to release this sadness."
- **Address Negative Self-Talk**: Negative self-beliefs, such as "I am not good enough" or "I will never get better," are common in depression. Using EFT to confront and reframe these thoughts can help to shift the individual's perception and alleviate feelings of worthlessness.
- **Use EFT for Physical Symptoms**: Tapping on acupressure points while focusing on physical symptoms of depression, such as low energy or muscle tension, can help to release the underlying emotional energy and restore balance to the body.
- **Practice Regularly**: Like any therapeutic technique, consistency is key. Regular tapping can help reinforce positive shifts in mood and help the individual stay grounded during difficult times.

Emotional Freedom Technique (EFT) offers a promising approach for those struggling with depression. By addressing both the emotional and physical aspects of the condition, EFT helps individuals reframe negative thought patterns, release emotional blockages, and alleviate the physical symptoms of depression. Through case studies and research, EFT has proven to be an effective complementary therapy for reducing depression symptoms and providing long-term relief. Whether used alongside traditional treatments or as a standalone method, EFT provides a powerful tool for those seeking a natural and holistic approach to mental well-being.

EFT for achieving emotional balance

Emotional imbalance can manifest in a variety of ways, from stress and anxiety to mood swings and feelings of overwhelm. These imbalances are often rooted in unresolved emotions, negative thought patterns, or past experiences that continue to influence one's emotional state. Achieving emotional balance involves recognizing and addressing these emotional disruptions, allowing individuals to regain control over their emotional responses and cultivate a sense of well-being. One of the most effective tools for this is the Emotional Freedom Technique (EFT), which works by addressing the root causes of emotional distress through a combination of acupressure and psychological techniques.

How EFT Promotes Emotional Balance

EFT operates on the principle that emotional distress is the result of blockages or disruptions in the body's energy system. When an individual experiences negative emotions, these feelings can create energetic blockages that interfere with the natural flow of energy. By tapping on specific acupressure points while focusing on the issue at hand, EFT helps release these blockages, restoring emotional and physical balance. This process is believed to recalibrate the body's energy system, allowing the person to feel calmer, more centered, and emotionally balanced.

The tapping points used in EFT correspond to meridian points that are traditionally associated with acupuncture. These points are thought to be connected to different areas of emotional and physical health. By tapping on these points while verbalizing specific emotional concerns, individuals can clear negative energy and allow positive emotions to flow more freely. This process helps individuals regain emotional equilibrium by breaking the cycle of stress, anxiety, and emotional reactivity.

Identifying Emotional Imbalances

Emotional imbalances often arise from unresolved trauma, chronic stress, negative self-talk, or repressed emotions. These imbalances can manifest as persistent feelings of anxiety, anger, sadness, or even physical symptoms like tension or fatigue. EFT works by helping individuals identify and address the specific emotional issues that are causing their distress. By focusing on these emotions during the tapping process, EFT encourages emotional release and promotes a more balanced state of mind.

For example, someone who struggles with chronic stress may feel on edge most of the time, with physical symptoms like tight shoulders, racing thoughts, and difficulty relaxing. These emotional and physical symptoms are often linked to unresolved feelings of fear, overwhelm, or insecurity. EFT helps by focusing on these emotional triggers and releasing their grip, leading to a reduction in physical tension and a sense of calm.

Releasing Negative Emotions with EFT

EFT is particularly effective at helping individuals release negative emotions that can create emotional imbalance. Common negative emotions such as fear, anger, guilt, shame, and sadness can be stored in the body, leading to long-term emotional disruption if not addressed. By tapping on the acupressure points while focusing on these emotions, EFT provides a direct and powerful way to release these trapped feelings.

For instance, if an individual is experiencing anger due to a past event, they may focus on the memory or the feelings of frustration while tapping on the points. The tapping process helps to neutralize the emotional charge associated with the memory, reducing the intensity of the emotion. As the person taps, they may find that the anger diminishes, leaving them with a greater sense of emotional balance and clarity.

EFT for Self-Acceptance and Emotional Regulation

One of the most powerful applications of EFT in achieving emotional balance is its ability to foster self-acceptance and emotional regulation. Many people experience emotional imbalance due to negative beliefs about themselves or an inability to manage their emotions effectively. EFT helps individuals confront these negative self-beliefs and develop healthier, more compassionate perspectives.

For example, someone who struggles with low self-esteem may use EFT to tap on feelings of unworthiness or inadequacy. By focusing on these beliefs and tapping through the points, the individual can reframe their perception of themselves and begin to accept their flaws and imperfections with greater kindness. Over time, this practice can lead to a more balanced emotional state, where the individual feels more at peace with themselves and their emotional experiences.

EFT also plays a role in improving emotional regulation, helping individuals learn how to respond to emotions in a balanced and constructive way. Instead of reacting impulsively to stressors, EFT helps individuals tap into their emotional responses and process them in a healthier manner. This enhances their ability to navigate life's challenges with resilience and composure.

EFT for Mood Swings and Emotional Overwhelm

Mood swings and emotional overwhelm can be particularly disruptive to emotional balance, often making it difficult for individuals to maintain a consistent sense of well-being. Whether these fluctuations are triggered by hormonal changes, life events, or stress, EFT can be a valuable tool for restoring emotional stability.

For instance, individuals who experience mood swings due to hormonal imbalances or premenstrual syndrome (PMS) can use EFT to help alleviate the emotional intensity of these swings. By tapping on the specific emotions tied to mood shifts—such as irritability, sadness, or anxiety—individuals can reduce the severity of their emotional ups and downs, allowing for a more balanced and stable emotional state.

Likewise, those who feel emotionally overwhelmed due to work, family, or personal challenges can use EFT to regain perspective and calm. By tapping through the emotional layers of overwhelm, individuals can release the pent-up stress and regain a sense of control and clarity.

Practical EFT Techniques for Emotional Balance

- **Tapping on Negative Emotions**: The first step in using EFT for emotional balance is to identify the specific negative emotion causing the imbalance. For example, if you're feeling anxious, your setup statement might be, "Even though I feel anxious about the future, I deeply and completely accept myself." As you tap through the points, focus on the physical and emotional sensations tied to your anxiety.
- **Reframing Negative Thoughts**: EFT is also effective at reframing negative thought patterns that contribute to emotional imbalances. If you're dealing with feelings of worthlessness, use a setup statement such as, "Even though I feel like I am not good enough, I choose to believe in my worth." Tapping while repeating these affirmations can help shift your perspective and restore emotional balance.
- **Daily Tapping Practice**: Regular EFT practice is key to maintaining emotional balance. By incorporating tapping into your daily routine, you can stay grounded and centered, reducing the buildup of stress and emotional tension. Use tapping as a preventative measure to keep your emotions in check and avoid the escalation of negative feelings.
- **Tapping for Relaxation**: EFT is also a powerful tool for promoting relaxation and relieving physical tension. If you're feeling overwhelmed or stressed, try tapping while focusing on deep breathing and relaxation. This can help release pent-up emotions and restore a sense of calm and emotional balance.

Emotional balance is essential for mental and physical well-being, and EFT provides a powerful tool for achieving and maintaining this balance. By addressing the root causes of emotional distress and using tapping to release negative emotions, individuals can restore harmony to their emotional state. Whether you're dealing with stress, mood swings, or long-standing emotional imbalances, EFT offers an effective and holistic approach to emotional healing. With consistent practice, EFT can help you achieve greater emotional resilience, self-acceptance, and overall well-being, allowing you to navigate life's challenges with greater ease and balance.

Applying EFT to alleviate depression

Depression is a multifaceted mental health condition that affects not only mood but also physical well-being, often manifesting as fatigue, sleep disturbances, and a sense of hopelessness. While traditional treatments such as medication and therapy are effective for many, Emotional Freedom Technique (EFT) has emerged as a complementary approach that can help alleviate depressive symptoms by addressing both the emotional and physiological aspects of the condition. EFT combines acupressure with cognitive techniques to clear emotional blockages, restore energy balance, and shift negative thought patterns, offering a promising tool for those dealing with depression.

How EFT Works to Alleviate Depression

At the core of EFT is the idea that emotional distress, including the deep sadness and negativity associated with depression, is often linked to imbalances or blockages in the body's energy system. These blockages are thought to result from unresolved emotions, past trauma, or negative beliefs. By tapping on specific acupressure points on the body while focusing on the issue causing emotional distress, EFT aims to release these blockages, allowing energy to flow freely and reducing the intensity of depressive symptoms.

Tapping on these meridian points (which are similar to those used in acupuncture) signals the brain to process the emotional experience differently. This helps to reduce the emotional charge tied to negative thoughts and traumatic memories, thus lowering the emotional intensity of depression and promoting a more balanced, calm state of mind.

Addressing Negative Thought Patterns

One of the hallmark features of depression is the constant cycle of negative thought patterns, such as feelings of worthlessness, guilt, and hopelessness. These thoughts can become self-perpetuating, reinforcing the depressive state and making it difficult for individuals to break free. EFT helps to disrupt this cycle by targeting the underlying emotional causes of these thoughts. By tapping while verbalizing statements like, "Even though I feel worthless, I deeply and completely accept myself," the individual is encouraged to confront and reframe these beliefs.

As the tapping continues, the intensity of these negative beliefs often decreases, allowing individuals to experience a shift in their perception of themselves and their situation. This process can help create a sense of self-compassion, acceptance, and empowerment—qualities that are essential for overcoming depression.

Releasing Emotional Blockages

Depression often stems from repressed or unresolved emotions—whether from past trauma, grief, or chronic stress. These unresolved feelings can become "stuck" in the body, contributing to feelings of emotional heaviness and disconnection. EFT provides a safe and gentle way to release these stored emotions. By focusing on specific memories, experiences, or feelings while tapping, individuals can begin to process and release the emotional charge associated with them.

For example, someone who is depressed due to unresolved grief might tap while focusing on the loss they experienced. As the tapping continues, the emotional intensity surrounding the grief may lessen, allowing the person to experience a greater sense of peace and emotional clarity. This emotional release helps to clear the mental fog that often accompanies depression, promoting a more balanced and stable emotional state.

EFT for Physical Symptoms of Depression

In addition to emotional symptoms, depression often manifests physically, with symptoms such as fatigue, muscle tension, changes in appetite, and disrupted sleep patterns. EFT can help alleviate these physical symptoms by tapping on the body's energy points while focusing on the physical sensations tied to depression. As individuals tap through the points, the physical tension in the body begins to release, leading to a reduction in fatigue, better sleep quality, and improved energy levels.

For example, if a person is experiencing tightness in their chest due to anxiety related to depression, they can tap on the acupressure points while focusing on that specific sensation. This can help to release the physical discomfort, thereby easing the associated emotional distress. By addressing both the physical and emotional symptoms of depression simultaneously, EFT offers a holistic approach to healing.

Case Studies and Evidence for EFT's Effectiveness

A number of studies and case reports have shown that EFT can be an effective tool for alleviating symptoms of depression. One study published in the *Journal of Nervous and Mental Disease* found that participants who underwent EFT treatment experienced significant reductions in depression, anxiety, and stress. The study also found that these improvements were sustained over time, suggesting that EFT may offer long-term benefits for individuals dealing with depression.

Another case study involved a woman named Maria, who had struggled with severe depression for over 10 years. Despite trying various forms of treatment, including medication and cognitive-behavioral therapy (CBT), Maria's symptoms persisted. After just a few EFT sessions focusing on her feelings of low self-worth and unresolved trauma, she reported a significant reduction in depressive symptoms. Her mood lifted, she experienced fewer feelings of hopelessness, and she began to reconnect with her passions. This case highlights the potential of EFT to help individuals address the underlying emotional causes of depression and achieve lasting relief.

Combining EFT with Traditional Treatment

While EFT can be a powerful standalone treatment for depression, it is often most effective when used in conjunction with traditional therapies such as medication or talk therapy. Many individuals find that combining EFT with these methods enhances the overall benefits. For instance, EFT can be used to complement the work done in therapy by addressing emotional triggers and reinforcing new, healthier thought patterns.

Additionally, EFT can be a valuable self-help tool, providing individuals with a technique they can use at home to manage their depression symptoms between therapy sessions. The ability to tap on their own, especially during moments of emotional distress, empowers individuals to take an active role in their healing process.

Practical Steps for Using EFT to Alleviate Depression

- **Identify the Emotion**: Begin by pinpointing the specific emotion or situation that is contributing to your depression. Focus on the core feelings, such as sadness, hopelessness, or anxiety.
- **Use a Setup Statement**: Formulate a setup statement to acknowledge the emotion while also expressing self-acceptance. For example, "Even though I feel hopeless and stuck, I deeply and completely accept myself."
- **Tap Through the Points**: While repeating the setup statement, tap on the acupressure points, starting at the top of the head and moving down to the collarbone and under the arms. Focus on the emotional sensations as you tap.
- **Reassess Your Feelings**: After completing a round of tapping, take a moment to assess the intensity of your depression. You may notice that your feelings have lessened, allowing for a sense of relief or clarity.
- **Repeat as Needed**: EFT is most effective when practiced regularly. If depressive feelings return, continue tapping on them, adjusting the setup statement as necessary. Over time, this can help reduce the emotional charge tied to depression.

EFT offers a powerful, non-invasive approach to alleviating depression by addressing both the emotional and physical aspects of the condition. Through tapping on acupressure points while focusing on negative emotions, past trauma, and physical symptoms, individuals can release emotional blockages, reframe negative thought patterns, and experience relief from the pervasive sadness associated with depression. With growing scientific support and numerous case studies demonstrating its effectiveness, EFT provides a promising tool for those seeking an alternative or complementary treatment for depression. By integrating EFT into a comprehensive treatment plan, individuals can achieve lasting emotional balance and improved well-being.

Examples and success stories

Emotional Freedom Technique (EFT) has been used by thousands of people worldwide to address a variety of emotional and psychological challenges, including stress, anxiety, trauma, and depression. Through tapping on specific acupressure points while focusing on emotional issues, EFT helps release blockages in the body's energy system, leading to relief and healing. Over the years, many success stories have emerged that highlight the transformative effects of this technique. These real-life examples provide insight into how EFT can offer lasting emotional relief and change.

Case Study 1: Overcoming Anxiety and Panic Attacks

Sarah, a 32-year-old woman, had struggled with chronic anxiety and panic attacks for years. Despite trying various therapies, including cognitive-behavioral therapy (CBT) and medication, she found only temporary relief. Her anxiety often escalated in social situations, and she felt trapped in a cycle of fear that severely impacted her personal and professional life. After learning about EFT from a therapist specializing in energy psychology, Sarah decided to give it a try.

During her first EFT session, Sarah tapped on the acupressure points while focusing on the specific fear she experienced in social settings. Her setup statement was, "Even though I feel terrified and anxious in social situations, I deeply and completely accept myself." Over the course of several sessions, Sarah's anxiety levels began to drop significantly. The panic attacks became less frequent, and she felt more confident engaging with others. She could not believe how much tapping had shifted her emotional responses, and she no longer felt as though she was a prisoner of her anxiety. Today, Sarah continues to use EFT whenever she feels anxious, and the technique has become a key tool in her mental health toolkit.

Case Study 2: Healing from Childhood Trauma

John, a 45-year-old man, had experienced emotional and physical abuse as a child. Although he had worked through some aspects of his trauma in therapy, he still carried significant emotional baggage that he could not seem to shake. He struggled with feelings of low self-worth, anger, and resentment that affected his relationships and daily life. His therapist recommended EFT as a complementary treatment to help release the emotional charge tied to his unresolved trauma.

In his EFT sessions, John tapped on memories of his childhood abuse and focused on the overwhelming emotions tied to those memories. His setup statements included, "Even though I feel angry about what happened to me as a child, I choose to release this anger and heal." Over time, John noticed a remarkable shift in his emotional state. The anger and resentment he had carried for decades began to dissipate, and he was able to view his past with more compassion and understanding. EFT helped him release the emotional blockages that had kept him stuck, and he found greater peace within himself. Today, John feels freer from the grip of his past trauma and has strengthened his relationships with family and friends.

Case Study 3: Alleviating Depression and Finding Hope

Maria, a 39-year-old woman, had been battling depression for several years. Despite trying medication and traditional therapy, she struggled with a sense of hopelessness and sadness that seemed to weigh her down. Her self-esteem was low, and she often felt overwhelmed by negative thoughts. When a friend recommended EFT, Maria was initially skeptical but decided to try it as a last resort.

Her EFT sessions focused on the intense sadness and feelings of unworthiness that she had carried for years. One of her common setup statements was, "Even though I feel like I'm not good enough and will never get better, I choose to love and accept myself." As Maria tapped through the acupressure points while addressing her emotional blocks, she noticed a gradual improvement in her mood. Over several weeks, her depression lifted, and she experienced moments of joy that had been absent for a long time. She reported feeling more hopeful, less burdened by negative thoughts, and more connected to her own sense of self-worth. EFT helped Maria challenge her limiting beliefs, and she continues to use the technique regularly to maintain her emotional well-being.

Case Study 4: Reducing Physical Pain and Emotional Stress

Tom, a 50-year-old man, had been dealing with chronic pain from a car accident he suffered several years ago. The pain was compounded by stress and frustration, as it limited his ability to participate in daily activities. Doctors had prescribed various treatments, but Tom still struggled with both the physical and emotional toll of his injury. A friend introduced him to EFT, and although Tom was initially doubtful, he decided to try tapping to see if it could provide any relief.

In his EFT sessions, Tom focused not only on the physical pain but also on the emotional stress surrounding the accident. His setup statements often included, "Even though I have this pain in my back and I feel frustrated and helpless, I choose to release the emotional charge and allow healing." As he tapped through the acupressure points, Tom began to notice a decrease in both his physical pain and emotional tension. His back pain lessened, and he found himself feeling calmer and more positive about his recovery. He continued to use EFT as part of his self-care routine, and over time, his pain management improved, along with his emotional resilience.

Case Study 5: Achieving Emotional Balance During High Stress

Rachel, a 28-year-old professional, worked in a high-stress corporate environment that demanded long hours and constant attention to detail. The pressure of deadlines and expectations caused Rachel to feel overwhelmed, anxious, and emotionally drained. She began to experience frequent bouts of stress-related headaches and difficulty sleeping. After hearing about EFT from a colleague, Rachel decided to try it as a tool for managing her stress.

During her EFT sessions, Rachel focused on the stress and anxiety she felt at work. Her setup statement was, "Even though I feel overwhelmed by my job and the pressure to perform, I deeply and completely accept myself." As she continued tapping, Rachel noticed a gradual reduction in her stress levels. She found that the headaches became less frequent, and she was able to manage her emotions more effectively. The tapping allowed her to process the underlying emotional tension that was contributing to her stress, leading to improved emotional balance and greater overall well-being.

These success stories highlight the transformative power of Emotional Freedom Technique in helping individuals overcome emotional and physical challenges. From alleviating anxiety and depression to healing from trauma and managing stress, EFT provides a versatile and effective approach to emotional healing. The common thread in these stories is the ability of EFT to address both the emotional and physical aspects of distress, offering a holistic solution that leads to lasting relief. As more people discover and use EFT, it continues to prove itself as a valuable tool for those seeking to improve their emotional well-being and achieve a balanced, healthy life.

Using EFT for Trauma and PTSD

Trauma and Post-Traumatic Stress Disorder (PTSD) are deeply impactful conditions, often leading to long-term emotional, physical, and psychological distress. Traditional treatments for trauma and PTSD, such as cognitive-behavioral therapy (CBT) and medication, can be effective for many individuals. However, Emotional Freedom Technique (EFT) has emerged as a complementary and, in some cases, transformative approach for healing trauma and alleviating PTSD symptoms. By addressing both the emotional and physiological components of trauma, EFT offers a holistic method of healing that targets the body's energy system, helping to release the emotional charge associated with traumatic memories.

Understanding the Emotional Impact of Trauma and PTSD

Trauma occurs when an individual experiences a deeply distressing event that overwhelms their ability to cope. This may include physical or emotional abuse, accidents, natural disasters, combat situations, or the sudden loss of a loved one. PTSD, a common outcome of trauma, is characterized by persistent symptoms such as flashbacks, nightmares, hypervigilance, and emotional numbness. These symptoms can disrupt daily life, leading to difficulties in relationships, work, and overall well-being.

At the core of both trauma and PTSD is the way in which the body and mind store the emotional charge tied to these distressing events. While the brain processes memories of the event, the body can "freeze" the emotional energy associated with that trauma, creating blockages that prevent healing. These blockages can lead to physical symptoms such as tension, pain, and fatigue, as well as emotional responses like anxiety, depression, and irritability.

How EFT Helps Heal Trauma and PTSD

EFT is based on the idea that unresolved emotions and traumatic experiences create imbalances in the body's energy system, leading to physical and emotional symptoms. By tapping on specific acupressure points while focusing on the traumatic memories or emotional distress, EFT aims to clear these blockages, restore energy flow, and reframe the emotional response to the trauma.

The process involves the individual tapping on the body's meridian points—such as the top of the head, eyebrow, under the eyes, and collarbone—while verbalizing specific thoughts or feelings related to the traumatic experience. This combination of physical stimulation and cognitive processing helps the brain to reprocess the trauma, reducing the intensity of the emotional charge and allowing the individual to view the memory without experiencing overwhelming emotional distress.

EFT for Releasing Trauma-Related Emotions

One of the primary benefits of EFT in trauma healing is its ability to target and release the intense emotions that are tied to traumatic memories. These emotions often manifest as anger, shame, fear, or sadness, and can lead to recurring thoughts or flashbacks that keep the individual emotionally stuck. Through tapping, EFT helps individuals confront these emotions in a controlled and safe environment, allowing them to process and release the emotional charge.

For example, an individual who has experienced a traumatic car accident may tap while focusing on the fear and helplessness they felt during the event. By repeating phrases such as, "Even though I feel terrified and helpless from the accident, I deeply and completely accept myself," they can start to reduce the intensity of the fear and trauma associated with the memory. As the tapping continues, the emotional distress attached to the memory may lessen, allowing the individual to recall the event with less emotional pain.

EFT for Processing Traumatic Memories

Traumatic memories are often stored in the brain as fragmented, highly emotional experiences. These memories may be difficult to process and can trigger flashbacks, panic attacks, or hyperarousal when triggered by reminders. EFT provides a method of processing these memories by focusing on the specific details of the trauma while tapping on the acupressure points.

For example, if someone has experienced combat-related trauma, they might revisit specific memories, such as the sounds, sights, or sensations that occurred during their time in the field. By tapping on the corresponding meridian points, the individual can release the intense emotional charge tied to these memories. This process helps to integrate the traumatic experience into the person's overall life narrative, reducing the impact it has on their emotional and mental health.

EFT for Reducing PTSD Symptoms

PTSD is characterized by persistent symptoms that interfere with daily life, including hypervigilance, intrusive thoughts, and emotional numbness. These symptoms often stem from unresolved trauma and the body's inability to process the emotional energy related to the traumatic event. EFT helps by addressing both the emotional and physical components of PTSD, leading to a reduction in symptom severity.

By tapping on specific acupressure points while focusing on PTSD-related triggers, such as flashbacks or feelings of helplessness, individuals can begin to reframe their emotional response to these triggers. EFT helps to desensitize the emotional charge associated with these triggers, allowing the individual to experience less anxiety, fear, and distress when reminded of the trauma. Over time, the frequency and intensity of PTSD symptoms may decrease, leading to improved emotional stability and a better quality of life.

Case Studies of EFT for Trauma and PTSD

Several case studies demonstrate the effectiveness of EFT in treating trauma and PTSD. In one study, a group of veterans with PTSD participated in EFT sessions over the course of several weeks. The results showed a significant reduction in PTSD symptoms, including a decrease in the frequency of flashbacks, hypervigilance, and sleep disturbances. Participants also reported improvements in overall mood and emotional regulation.

In another case, a woman named Lisa had experienced sexual abuse as a child. For years, she struggled with low self-esteem, anxiety, and flashbacks to the abuse. After several EFT sessions focused on the trauma, Lisa reported that her flashbacks decreased significantly, and she no longer felt triggered by reminders of the abuse. She felt empowered to move forward in her life, using EFT as a tool to manage any emotional distress that arose.

EFT as Part of a Comprehensive Healing Approach

While EFT can be an effective stand-alone therapy for trauma and PTSD, it is often most beneficial when used as part of a comprehensive healing plan. For some individuals, combining EFT with other therapies, such as talk therapy, mindfulness practices, or bodywork, can provide additional layers of support. EFT can complement these approaches by offering a rapid way to release emotional blockages and reframe negative thought patterns.

Additionally, EFT is a versatile tool that can be used both in a therapeutic setting and as a self-help practice. Many individuals who experience trauma or PTSD find that learning EFT allows them to continue their healing process at home, helping them to manage stress and anxiety between therapy sessions.

EFT offers a powerful, effective, and non-invasive approach to healing trauma and alleviating PTSD symptoms. By addressing both the emotional and physical aspects of trauma, EFT helps to release the blockages that prevent healing, allowing individuals to process their traumatic experiences without being overwhelmed by emotional distress. Through tapping on specific acupressure points while focusing on the trauma-related emotions and memories, individuals can experience lasting relief from PTSD symptoms and reclaim their emotional well-being. With a growing body of evidence and numerous success stories, EFT is becoming a valuable tool for those seeking healing from trauma and PTSD, providing a holistic and empowering approach to recovery.

How EFT can help trauma survivors

Trauma survivors often carry deep emotional wounds that can manifest in various ways, from anxiety and depression to physical symptoms such as chronic pain or insomnia. Healing from trauma is a complex process, but Emotional Freedom Technique (EFT) has emerged as an effective tool for helping individuals release the emotional charge associated with their traumatic experiences. EFT works by tapping on specific acupressure points on the body while focusing on the emotions tied to the trauma. This combination of physical stimulation and emotional processing helps to clear blockages in the body's energy system, leading to emotional relief and healing.

EFT as a Trauma Recovery Tool

Trauma can overwhelm the body's ability to process emotions, often leading to stored emotional energy that results in distressing symptoms like flashbacks, hypervigilance, and emotional numbness. In some cases, this energy becomes "stuck" in the body, manifesting as physical tension, pain, or illnesses. EFT helps trauma survivors by reprogramming the body's emotional response to these experiences, allowing them to process the trauma in a healthier, more balanced way.

Unlike traditional talk therapies, which often require verbalizing traumatic memories in great detail, EFT uses a gentle approach that combines tapping on acupressure points with verbal affirmations focused on the trauma. This process helps to clear the emotional residue without the need to relive the trauma in a highly emotional way. This can make EFT particularly beneficial for those who find it difficult or retraumatizing to talk about their past experiences in detail.

Releasing Emotional Blocks Tied to Trauma

One of the most powerful aspects of EFT for trauma survivors is its ability to help them release the emotional blocks that are tied to their traumatic memories. These blocks may consist of intense feelings of fear, shame, anger, or helplessness, all of which are common responses to traumatic events. Tapping on specific acupressure points while focusing on these emotions can help clear the energetic blockages associated with the trauma, reducing the intensity of the emotional response.

For example, a trauma survivor may have a heightened emotional reaction when reminded of the traumatic event, such as feeling paralyzed by fear or overwhelmed by anger. Using EFT, they can focus on the specific emotions that arise when thinking about the trauma and tap through the meridian points, gradually reducing the emotional intensity. Over time, this process can help trauma survivors gain a sense of emotional release, calm, and control over their responses to traumatic memories.

Reprogramming the Body's Stress Response

The body's natural response to trauma is often a state of heightened stress, where the fight-or-flight response is activated. For many trauma survivors, this chronic state of stress can lead to long-term physical and emotional issues such as anxiety, sleep disturbances, and heightened sensitivity to stressors. EFT helps to reprogram the body's stress response by signaling to the brain that the trauma is no longer an immediate threat, allowing the body to relax and return to a state of emotional balance.

As trauma survivors tap on specific acupressure points, they send signals to the brain that help regulate the body's autonomic nervous system. This can help reduce the body's fight-or-flight response, leading to a decrease in anxiety and stress. Over time, the individual's nervous system becomes less reactive to trauma-related triggers, making it easier to manage everyday stress and emotional challenges.

Enhancing Self-Compassion and Acceptance

Trauma survivors often struggle with feelings of shame, guilt, or self-blame, which can be barriers to healing. These feelings can distort an individual's self-image, making it difficult to move forward. EFT offers a way to address these negative self-beliefs by incorporating self-acceptance and compassion into the tapping process. By using statements such as, "Even though I feel ashamed of what happened, I choose to love and accept myself," EFT helps to promote healing and self-compassion.

This focus on self-acceptance can be particularly powerful for survivors of childhood abuse, sexual assault, or other forms of interpersonal trauma, where the individual may have internalized feelings of worthlessness or undesirability. EFT helps trauma survivors reframe these beliefs, fostering a more positive self-image and empowering them to heal.

Trauma Recovery in Stages

EFT can be used to address trauma in stages, allowing individuals to process different aspects of their traumatic experiences over time. For example, a trauma survivor may first focus on the emotional aspects of the trauma, tapping through feelings of fear, sadness, or anger. Once these emotions have been processed, the individual can work on physical symptoms associated with the trauma, such as pain or tension. In some cases, EFT can also be used to help survivors reframe negative thought patterns or beliefs that have formed as a result of the trauma, such as beliefs about their safety, worth, or ability to trust others.

This staged approach allows survivors to work at their own pace, addressing the most pressing emotional or physical symptoms first and gradually moving toward deeper levels of healing. The ability to break down the trauma recovery process into manageable steps makes EFT particularly effective for individuals who may feel overwhelmed by the magnitude of their healing journey.

Case Studies of EFT and Trauma Recovery

Numerous case studies have demonstrated the effectiveness of EFT for trauma recovery. For instance, a woman who survived a car accident that left her with both physical injuries and emotional scars found relief through EFT. Initially, she struggled with feelings of anxiety, nightmares, and physical pain related to the accident. After a few EFT sessions focusing on the emotional charge tied to the event, she reported a significant reduction in her anxiety and physical pain. She also found that her nightmares became less frequent, and she could recall the event with less emotional distress.

Another example involves a combat veteran suffering from PTSD. He had experienced repeated nightmares, intrusive thoughts, and emotional numbness, which had made it difficult for him to connect with his family and live a fulfilling life. After several EFT sessions, focusing on specific memories related to his combat experiences, the veteran reported a significant reduction in flashbacks and intrusive thoughts. He also found it easier to reconnect with his emotions and engage more fully in daily activities.

Benefits of EFT for Trauma Survivors

1. **Emotional Regulation:** EFT helps trauma survivors regulate intense emotions such as fear, anger, and shame by clearing the emotional charge associated with trauma-related memories.
2. **Physical Healing:** EFT can help reduce physical symptoms of trauma, such as pain, tension, and sleep disturbances, by addressing the body's stress response.
3. **Empowerment and Self-Acceptance:** EFT promotes feelings of self-compassion and acceptance, helping individuals heal their self-image and rebuild their sense of worth.
4. **Holistic Approach:** EFT works on both the emotional and physical levels, providing a holistic method of healing that addresses the interconnectedness of body, mind, and energy.
5. **Self-Sufficiency:** Trauma survivors can learn to use EFT on their own, making it a valuable tool for self-care and ongoing emotional support.

EFT offers a gentle, effective, and empowering method for trauma survivors to process and heal from their experiences. By releasing emotional blocks, reprogramming the body's stress response, and enhancing self-compassion, EFT helps individuals recover from trauma in a way that is holistic and sustainable. Through its combination of acupressure and emotional processing, EFT enables survivors to regain a sense of control, peace, and emotional balance, allowing them to move forward in their healing journey. Whether used in conjunction with other therapies or as a stand-alone practice, EFT offers a valuable tool for trauma recovery.

Techniques for addressing trauma with EFT

Addressing trauma with Emotional Freedom Technique (EFT) involves a combination of tapping on specific acupressure points while focusing on the emotional distress tied to the traumatic experience. This unique method helps trauma survivors process their emotional reactions and reprogram their body's stress responses. The process can be tailored to suit individual needs, providing a customizable and effective approach to healing. Several techniques within EFT can be particularly useful when working through trauma, allowing individuals to release stored emotional energy and regain a sense of emotional balance and well-being.

1. Basic EFT Tapping Sequence

The core of EFT involves tapping on specific points along the body's meridians while focusing on the negative emotion or physical symptom associated with the trauma. The typical tapping sequence begins with the karate chop point (on the side of the hand), followed by the other key meridian points:

- Top of the head (Crown point)
- Eyebrow (at the beginning of the eyebrow, near the nose)
- Side of the eye (at the bone at the outer corner of the eye)
- Under the eye (on the bone beneath the eye)
- Under the nose (between the nose and upper lip)
- Chin point (below the lower lip)
- Collarbone (just below the collarbone, about an inch from the center)
- Under the arm (about 4 inches below the armpit)

As you tap on these points, you focus on the trauma, verbalizing a setup statement (e.g., "Even though I feel scared about the accident, I deeply and completely accept myself") and following up with reminder phrases that reflect your emotional experience (e.g., "This fear from the car crash").

The tapping helps to release the intensity of the emotions tied to the trauma and restores a sense of calm by activating the body's energy system. Over time, this technique can reduce emotional charge and reframe the trauma in a way that it no longer triggers overwhelming emotional responses.

2. The Movie Technique

The "Movie Technique" is a particularly useful tool for survivors of trauma who may find it difficult to directly confront the trauma or talk about it in detail. This technique involves imagining the traumatic event as if it were a scene in a movie or watching it on a screen. By mentally "replaying" the traumatic event from a detached perspective, individuals can reduce the emotional intensity that comes with vividly remembering the experience.

While visualizing the traumatic event as a "movie," you would begin tapping through the EFT sequence. As you tap, you gradually notice that the emotional intensity of the memory begins to decrease. This detachment allows individuals to reframe their relationship with the trauma and helps them confront it in a safe and controlled way. The Movie Technique is especially effective for individuals with deep-seated trauma who might struggle to speak directly about the event but can still access the emotional material through visualization.

3. The Tell the Story Technique

The "Tell the Story" technique is especially helpful for those who are ready to process their trauma in more detail. In this method, the individual recounts their traumatic experience, either silently or aloud, while tapping through the meridian points. The focus is on expressing the emotions, thoughts, and physical sensations associated with the event.

As the person taps through the sequence, they continue telling their story, repeating the setup statement ("Even though I feel overwhelmed by this memory, I deeply accept myself") and the reminder phrases ("This fear from the past"). This technique helps to disarm the emotional charge by allowing the person to process the event without being emotionally overwhelmed. By tapping as they recount the trauma, the person can gradually desensitize their emotional and physical responses to the event, leading to emotional release and healing.

4. The Personal Peace Procedure

For individuals dealing with multiple layers of trauma or past emotional wounds, the "Personal Peace Procedure" is a more comprehensive method. In this approach, you write down a list of all the events, memories, and emotional issues that may be contributing to your overall sense of distress. This could include specific traumatic events, negative beliefs, or repressed emotions.

Once the list is created, you begin tapping on each issue individually, using the setup statement ("Even though I feel sadness about this memory, I accept myself") and tapping through the meridian points. The idea is to work through each memory or emotion on the list until you no longer feel emotionally charged by it. This method can be particularly effective for trauma survivors who have experienced complex or ongoing traumatic experiences that have built up over time.

The Personal Peace Procedure can be used as a regular self-help tool, helping trauma survivors to address old wounds and release emotional baggage. It also fosters emotional clarity and the ability to move forward without being bogged down by unresolved emotional issues.

5. Using EFT for Physical Trauma Symptoms

Trauma doesn't only affect emotions; it can also leave physical imprints, such as pain, tension, and fatigue. EFT can be particularly effective for addressing the physical aspects of trauma by tapping on both emotional memories and the physical sensations that are stored in the body.

For example, a person who has experienced a physical injury or accident may continue to feel pain or tension even after the injury has healed. This is often because the emotional stress of the trauma gets stored in the body. By tapping on the meridian points while focusing on the physical pain or discomfort, the individual can help release the emotional charge associated with the injury and reduce the pain sensation.

The physical symptoms may gradually subside as the body's energy system is restored to balance, helping the individual to heal both emotionally and physically from the trauma.

6. EFT for Reframing Negative Beliefs

Many trauma survivors develop negative core beliefs as a result of their traumatic experiences. These beliefs might include thoughts such as "I am not safe," "I am unworthy," or "I can't trust anyone." These limiting beliefs can keep individuals stuck in their trauma and prevent them from fully healing. EFT is effective in helping to identify and reframe these beliefs.

To address negative beliefs, the individual first taps through the meridian points while focusing on the belief ("Even though I feel unsafe, I choose to feel safe now"). After clearing the negative belief, the individual then taps on a positive affirmation, such as "I am safe," "I trust myself," or "I am worthy of love and happiness." This process helps to shift the individual's mindset, replacing limiting beliefs with healthier, empowering ones. Over time, this process can lead to a significant shift in the individual's sense of self-worth, safety, and confidence.

7. The Inner Child Technique

Many trauma survivors carry unresolved emotional pain from childhood or early life. The "Inner Child" technique helps individuals reconnect with the younger part of themselves that experienced the trauma. By using EFT to tap on issues related to the inner child—such as feelings of abandonment, neglect, or fear—the individual can begin to heal these wounds.

In this technique, the individual might focus on a specific childhood memory or emotion, tapping through the meridian points while offering words of comfort and reassurance to their inner child. This can be a deeply healing process, as it allows the person to offer the compassion and support they may not have received during the traumatic event. The Inner Child technique fosters self-compassion and helps to integrate the wounded parts of the self, allowing for healing and emotional growth.

The techniques for addressing trauma with EFT are varied and adaptable, allowing trauma survivors to find the approach that best suits their individual needs. Whether focusing on specific memories, reframing negative beliefs, or releasing physical pain, EFT offers a powerful way to process and heal from trauma. By tapping on acupressure points while targeting the emotional charge tied to the trauma, individuals can gradually reduce the intensity of their distress and reclaim a sense of peace and emotional balance. These techniques offer trauma survivors the opportunity to break free from the past, heal deep wounds, and move forward with greater emotional freedom.

Real case studies

EFT has shown promise in addressing a wide range of emotional and psychological challenges, from anxiety and depression to trauma and chronic pain. Real-life case studies highlight how this therapeutic technique can provide lasting relief, emotional healing, and a sense of empowerment. Below are some compelling examples of individuals who have experienced significant improvements through EFT.

1. Overcoming Trauma After a Car Accident

One case involved a woman named Sarah, who had been in a serious car accident. Although her physical injuries healed, she continued to suffer from anxiety, nightmares, and emotional numbness. The trauma left her feeling hypervigilant and fearful of driving, and she often found herself reliving the accident in her mind.

Sarah decided to try EFT after hearing about its potential benefits for trauma recovery. During her first session, she focused on the anxiety and fear associated with driving. While tapping on the meridian points, she verbalized her feelings: "Even though I feel scared when I get in the car, I accept myself and my fear." Over several sessions, Sarah also tapped through specific memories of the crash, beginning with the emotional charge she felt immediately after the accident and working through the overwhelming fear that accompanied her recovery.

As Sarah continued tapping on her fears and re-living the traumatic event in a more controlled way, her emotional response began to lessen. She reported that her nightmares became less frequent, and the anxiety she felt while driving gradually diminished. Within a few months, Sarah felt safe enough to drive again and no longer experienced the intense emotional triggers that had initially made the idea of getting behind the wheel unbearable.

2. Healing from Childhood Abuse

Mark, a man in his 40s, had struggled with feelings of shame, worthlessness, and anger due to a history of childhood abuse. Despite years of traditional therapy, Mark had a difficult time overcoming these deeply ingrained emotional wounds. The shame from his childhood had led him to self-destructive behavior, including substance abuse and relationship difficulties.

After hearing about EFT from a friend, Mark decided to give it a try. In his first EFT session, he focused on a memory from his childhood where he felt humiliated and abandoned by his parents. Mark tapped through the meridian points while saying: "Even though I feel ashamed about what happened, I choose to release this shame and accept myself."

Over time, Mark's sessions included tapping on a range of memories from his past, including times when he had been mistreated or abandoned. He also worked on reframing his negative beliefs about himself. "I am worthy of love and respect," he would affirm while tapping. As he continued with EFT, Mark noticed a shift in his self-image. He began to let go of the heavy emotional charge tied to his past and started feeling more self-compassion.

Six months later, Mark reported feeling a newfound sense of inner peace. His relationships improved, and he was able to reduce his reliance on substances. EFT had helped him process his trauma in a gentle and manageable way, allowing him to make positive changes in his life.

3. Dealing with Public Speaking Anxiety

Jane, a corporate professional, had struggled with debilitating anxiety about public speaking for most of her life. The thought of speaking in front of an audience would make her stomach churn, and she often experienced panic attacks before presentations. This anxiety started to affect her career, as she would avoid opportunities that required speaking in public or delivering presentations.

After hearing a colleague discuss the benefits of EFT, Jane decided to try it as a way to overcome her anxiety. In her first session, she focused on the overwhelming fear and dread she felt before presentations. "Even though I feel terrified of speaking in front of others, I choose to feel calm and confident," she would say while tapping through the meridian points.

After several EFT sessions, Jane began to notice a significant reduction in her anxiety. The physical symptoms of fear, like a racing heart and shallow breathing, were no longer as intense. Jane also worked on reframing her beliefs about speaking, focusing on positive affirmations like "I am a confident speaker," and "I can handle this situation with ease." By tapping before each presentation, she started feeling more in control and less anxious.

Six months after beginning EFT, Jane successfully delivered a high-stakes presentation to an audience of over 100 people without experiencing the panic attacks that once plagued her. She continued using EFT to manage stress and maintain her newfound confidence in public speaking.

4. Reducing Chronic Pain Linked to Trauma

Lena, a 55-year-old woman, had suffered from chronic neck and back pain for years. The pain began after a car accident, but despite physical therapy and pain medication, she continued to experience severe discomfort. Additionally, the pain was accompanied by anxiety, especially during flare-ups, and Lena suspected that her emotional state was contributing to the physical symptoms.

Lena's EFT practitioner helped her explore the connection between her physical pain and the unresolved emotions surrounding her accident. During her sessions, Lena tapped through the meridian points while focusing on both the emotional and physical pain. She would say: "Even though I still feel the pain from the accident, I choose to release this tension and allow my body to heal."

As Lena continued with EFT, she started to notice a gradual reduction in her pain levels. The anxiety that accompanied the flare-ups also decreased, and Lena found herself more able to relax during moments of discomfort. She continued to tap regularly on both the physical and emotional aspects of her pain, and within a few months, she reported that her pain had decreased by over 50%, allowing her to resume activities that had previously been impossible.

5. Relieving PTSD Symptoms After Combat

John, a military veteran, had been struggling with Post-Traumatic Stress Disorder (PTSD) after serving in a combat zone. He experienced recurring flashbacks, nightmares, hypervigilance, and feelings of detachment from others. Despite undergoing years of therapy, he still found it difficult to manage the intense emotions tied to his experiences.

After learning about EFT, John worked with a practitioner to address his PTSD symptoms. The focus of his sessions was to work through his traumatic memories in a way that was both safe and controlled. John began by tapping on the initial emotions that arose when thinking about his time in combat—fear, sadness, and anger. He used the setup phrase: "Even though I have these painful memories, I choose to release them and feel at peace."

Gradually, John began to feel more grounded and less triggered by flashbacks and intrusive thoughts. By continuing with EFT, he was able to tap on the emotions surrounding specific traumatic memories, allowing him to process them in a way that reduced their emotional charge. His nightmares became less frequent, and he reported feeling more present and connected with others.

A year after starting EFT, John had significant improvement in managing his PTSD symptoms. He was able to engage more fully in his life, enjoying moments with his family and pursuing new interests without being overwhelmed by the emotional residue of his combat experiences.

These case studies underscore the diverse ways in which EFT can provide emotional relief and healing. Whether addressing trauma, anxiety, pain, or self-esteem issues, the technique helps individuals break free from the grip of past experiences, reducing emotional distress and creating space for lasting positive change. The results experienced by Sarah, Mark, Jane, Lena, and John illustrate EFT's potential as a powerful tool in transforming emotional and physical well-being. As more people discover the benefits of this technique, it is clear that EFT offers a promising path to healing, one tapping session at a time.

EFT and Addiction

Addiction is a complex condition, often tied to both physical dependency and deep emotional pain. Whether the addiction is to substances like alcohol, drugs, nicotine, or behaviors such as gambling, food, or even technology, the cycle of cravings, compulsions, and emotional triggers can be overwhelming. Emotional Freedom Technique (EFT) has emerged as a powerful tool in breaking the patterns associated with addiction, offering a holistic approach to both the emotional and physical aspects of the problem. By using tapping on specific acupressure points while addressing the underlying emotional triggers, EFT helps individuals regain control over their habits and begin the process of recovery.

How EFT Helps with Addiction

Addiction is often driven by unresolved emotional issues such as trauma, stress, or negative core beliefs. Many people turn to substances or behaviors as a way to numb their emotions or cope with overwhelming feelings. EFT addresses these root emotional causes by targeting the psychological and emotional aspects of addiction, reducing cravings and restoring emotional balance. Here's how EFT works in addiction recovery:

1. **Emotional Root of Addiction:** Many individuals struggling with addiction are using substances or behaviors as a form of self-medication. This self-medication may be in response to past trauma, feelings of anxiety, depression, or low self-worth. EFT targets these emotional roots by helping individuals confront and release the negative emotions tied to their addiction. By tapping on specific acupressure points, the body's energy system is rebalanced, allowing for a reduction in emotional stress and a shift in the emotional triggers that drive the addictive behavior.
2. **Reducing Cravings and Urges:** One of the most immediate benefits of EFT is its ability to reduce cravings and compulsive urges. As individuals tap through the meridian points, they focus on the desire to use the substance or engage in the addictive behavior, repeating setup phrases like: "Even though I feel this overwhelming urge to drink, I choose to release this craving and feel calm." The tapping process sends signals to the brain that reduce the intensity of the craving, helping individuals regain control over their impulses.
3. **Changing Negative Beliefs:** Addiction is often fueled by negative beliefs, such as "I'm not good enough" or "I don't deserve to be happy." These beliefs may have developed early in life and have been reinforced by experiences of failure,

rejection, or trauma. EFT works to identify and reframe these beliefs by tapping while focusing on the limiting thoughts that underlie the addiction. Through consistent use of EFT, individuals can replace negative thought patterns with healthier, more empowering beliefs. This shift in mindset helps individuals view themselves as capable of change and worthy of recovery.

4. **Emotional Regulation and Stress Relief:** Many people turn to addictive substances or behaviors as a way to manage stress and emotional discomfort. EFT helps regulate the body's stress response by tapping on specific acupressure points that correspond to energy pathways in the body. By calming the nervous system, EFT enables individuals to process difficult emotions without resorting to their addictive behaviors. Over time, this ability to manage stress naturally leads to a reduction in the need for substances or behaviors that were once used as coping mechanisms.

5. **Breaking the Cycle of Relapse:** Addiction recovery is often marked by cycles of abstinence and relapse. After a period of sobriety, many individuals face intense emotional triggers that lead them back to their addictive habits. EFT can be a powerful tool in breaking these cycles by addressing the underlying emotional patterns that drive relapse. By tapping on past triggers, feelings of shame, or stress, individuals can desensitize themselves to the situations that might otherwise lead to a relapse. This allows them to create new emotional responses and healthier coping strategies.

EFT Techniques for Addiction Recovery

There are several EFT techniques that can be particularly useful for individuals working through addiction:

1. **The Craving Technique:** This technique is designed to reduce the intensity of cravings. The individual focuses on the specific craving they are experiencing (e.g., a desire for a cigarette, alcohol, or food) and taps through the meridian points while repeating a setup phrase like, "Even though I crave this substance, I choose to release this craving and feel at peace." By focusing on the physical sensations of the craving and tapping on the meridian points, the brain's association between the craving and the need for the substance weakens, allowing the individual to move past the desire.

2. **The Trauma or Emotional Root Technique:** Addiction is often linked to past trauma or unresolved emotional pain. In this technique, the individual focuses on the traumatic experience or emotion that may be contributing to the addiction. By tapping through the meridian points while thinking about the specific memory or emotion, the intensity of the emotional response is reduced. This technique helps the individual to process the underlying pain and create new, healthier emotional associations, reducing the need to turn to the addiction for relief.

3. **The Reframing Technique:** The individual focuses on the negative beliefs that contribute to the addiction (e.g., "I can't handle life without alcohol" or "I'm not worthy of recovery"). As they tap, they repeat positive affirmations like, "I am worthy of a healthy life," or "I can handle this challenge with ease." This helps to shift the individual's mindset from one of helplessness to empowerment, making it easier to let go of the addiction.
4. **The Future Pacing Technique:** After reducing cravings and processing emotional triggers, EFT can be used to visualize a future without addiction. The individual imagines themselves living a life free from addiction, experiencing the positive emotions associated with sobriety, and tapping through the meridian points while reinforcing their positive visualizations. This technique helps to solidify the individual's belief in their ability to live without addiction and prepares them mentally for the challenges ahead.

Real-World Case Studies

1. **Case Study: Alcohol Addiction Recovery**

John, a 40-year-old man, struggled with alcohol addiction for over 15 years. Despite trying multiple rehabilitation programs, he found it difficult to break the cycle of drinking. He would often turn to alcohol during moments of stress or when dealing with unresolved anger from past relationships. After learning about EFT, John decided to give it a try.

In his first EFT session, John tapped on the emotional triggers that led to his cravings, such as his unresolved anger and feelings of inadequacy. As he tapped, he focused on the specific urge to drink and repeated the affirmation, "Even though I feel the need to drink to escape my emotions, I choose to release this urge and feel calm."

After several weeks of using EFT daily, John noticed that his cravings decreased significantly. He no longer felt the overwhelming need to drink during stressful moments, and he was able to manage his emotions more effectively. Through continued use of EFT, John eventually became sober and was able to maintain his sobriety without the intense emotional urges that had once controlled his life.

2. **Case Study: Smoking Cessation**

Emily had been smoking for over a decade and had tried quitting multiple times without success. Each time she tried to quit, she would experience intense cravings and feelings of anxiety. She decided to try EFT after hearing about its benefits for breaking addictive behaviors.

During her sessions, Emily focused on the physical sensation of the craving and the emotional discomfort that triggered her urge to smoke. She tapped through the meridian points while repeating statements like, "Even though I feel this strong urge to smoke, I choose to release this craving and feel relaxed." Gradually, the intensity of the cravings reduced, and Emily no longer felt compelled to reach for a cigarette in stressful situations.

Within two months of practicing EFT, Emily was able to quit smoking entirely. She continued to use EFT to reinforce her commitment to staying smoke-free and to manage any lingering urges.

EFT offers a unique and effective approach to addiction recovery by addressing both the emotional and physical components of addiction. By tapping on acupressure points while focusing on cravings, emotional triggers, and limiting beliefs, individuals can break free from the cycles of addiction and create lasting change. Whether overcoming substance abuse, food addiction, or other compulsive behaviors, EFT provides a powerful tool for emotional healing, self-empowerment, and long-term recovery. The growing number of success stories speaks to the effectiveness of this holistic approach in helping individuals reclaim their lives and find freedom from addiction.

Using EFT to combat addiction

Addiction is a multifaceted condition that involves both physical dependence and deep-rooted emotional challenges. Whether it's addiction to substances like alcohol or drugs, or behavioral addictions such as gambling or food, the cycle of cravings and compulsions can feel inescapable. Emotional Freedom Technique (EFT) has emerged as a promising tool for combating addiction by addressing not only the physical aspects of dependency but also the emotional triggers and psychological roots that fuel addictive behaviors.

How EFT Works to Combat Addiction

Addiction often stems from the need to cope with unresolved emotions such as trauma, stress, anxiety, or low self-worth. Substances or behaviors that lead to addiction typically provide temporary relief, which reinforces the cycle of use. EFT helps break this cycle by targeting the emotional causes behind the addiction and providing individuals with healthier ways to process and manage their emotions. The tapping process uses acupressure points on the body to activate the body's energy system, which can help restore emotional balance and reduce cravings.

1. **Targeting Emotional Triggers:** Addiction is often triggered by strong emotions, whether it's anxiety, fear, sadness, or even boredom. EFT helps individuals identify and process these emotional triggers by tapping on specific acupressure points while focusing on the negative feelings or memories associated with their addiction. By addressing these emotions in a safe and controlled way, EFT helps individuals reduce the emotional charge tied to the addiction, making it easier to resist the urge to engage in the addictive behavior.
2. **Reducing Cravings and Urges:** One of the most immediate benefits of EFT in addiction recovery is its ability to reduce cravings. By tapping through meridian points while focusing on the craving itself, EFT helps diminish the intensity of the desire to engage in addictive behaviors. For example, an individual struggling with a smoking addiction may tap while focusing on the overwhelming urge to smoke, saying, "Even though I feel the need to smoke right now, I choose to release this craving and feel calm." This technique helps to weaken the connection between the craving and the need for the substance or behavior, making it easier to resist.
3. **Changing Negative Beliefs:** Many individuals with addiction hold limiting beliefs about themselves that contribute to their addictive behavior. Beliefs like "I'm not good enough" or "I don't deserve to be happy" can keep someone trapped in a cycle of self-destructive behavior. EFT can help individuals challenge and reframe

these negative beliefs by tapping on the emotional responses tied to them. Through this process, individuals can replace harmful beliefs with more positive, empowering ones, which supports the recovery process.

4. **Emotional Regulation:** Addiction often serves as a way of self-medicating emotional pain or discomfort. Over time, individuals become conditioned to reach for substances or behaviors as a way to numb or escape their feelings. EFT helps restore emotional regulation by tapping on meridian points associated with the body's energy system, which can soothe the nervous system and reduce the intensity of negative emotions. This process helps individuals develop healthier coping mechanisms and emotional resilience, reducing the need to rely on substances or behaviors for relief.

5. **Breaking the Cycle of Relapse:** Addiction recovery is often a process of progress and setbacks. Many individuals experience periods of sobriety followed by relapses, which can feel discouraging. EFT can help break the cycle of relapse by addressing the emotional triggers and stressors that lead to a return to addictive behaviors. By tapping on specific memories, fears, or past experiences, individuals can desensitize themselves to these emotional triggers, making it easier to stay on track with their recovery and avoid relapse.

EFT Techniques for Addiction Recovery

Several specific EFT techniques are particularly useful in combating addiction:

1. **Craving Reduction Technique:** This technique focuses on reducing the intensity of cravings. The individual taps on the meridian points while focusing on the craving itself. They may repeat a phrase like, "Even though I have this strong craving for [substance/behavior], I choose to release it now and feel calm." This tapping sequence helps weaken the craving and makes it easier to resist the temptation.

2. **The Emotional Root Technique:** Often, addiction is driven by deep emotional pain or trauma. This technique involves tapping on the emotional root causes of the addiction, such as past trauma, stress, or unresolved feelings. The individual may tap while focusing on specific memories or emotions, saying something like, "Even though I feel [emotion] because of [event], I choose to release this emotional burden and allow myself to heal." This technique helps to clear the emotional baggage that fuels the addiction.

3. **The Reframing Technique:** Negative beliefs about oneself can contribute to the cycle of addiction. The reframing technique involves tapping while focusing on these beliefs, such as, "I'm not worthy" or "I can't handle life without [substance]." While tapping, the individual repeats more positive affirmations like, "I am worthy of a healthy life" or "I am capable of overcoming this addiction." This technique helps to change the mental framework that supports the addiction, replacing it with empowering thoughts and beliefs.

4. **The Stress Relief Technique:** Since addiction is often a way of coping with stress, tapping for stress relief can help individuals manage their emotional responses. By focusing on the feeling of stress and tapping through the points, individuals can reduce anxiety, tension, and other stress-related emotions that may drive them to use substances or engage in addictive behaviors.
5. **The Future Pacing Technique:** Future pacing is a visualization technique that helps individuals imagine themselves free from addiction. By tapping while visualizing a future where they are living a healthy, addiction-free life, individuals can strengthen their commitment to recovery. This technique helps reinforce the belief that recovery is possible and encourages the individual to take positive action toward their goals.

Numerous success stories have highlighted the effectiveness of EFT in addiction recovery. Below are a few examples of how EFT has been applied to different types of addiction:

1. **Overcoming Alcohol Addiction:**

John, a 45-year-old man who had struggled with alcohol dependency for years, turned to EFT after realizing traditional treatments weren't enough. During his EFT sessions, John tapped on the emotional triggers that caused him to drink, such as stress at work and unresolved feelings of inadequacy. By using the craving reduction technique and focusing on his negative beliefs about himself, John noticed a significant decrease in his urge to drink. Over the course of several months, he found himself drinking less frequently, eventually achieving sobriety. He continued to use EFT regularly to reinforce his commitment to living an alcohol-free life.

2. **Breaking Free from Gambling Addiction:**

Sarah, a 30-year-old woman, had been struggling with a gambling addiction that was negatively impacting her finances and relationships. She began using EFT to address the emotional triggers behind her behavior, such as feelings of boredom and low self-esteem. By tapping on the urges to gamble and focusing on her desire to fill the emotional void, Sarah was able to break the cycle of compulsive gambling. Over time, she developed healthier ways to cope with her emotions and reduced her desire to gamble. EFT became a key part of her recovery process, helping her rebuild her life and relationships.

3. **Cigarette Smoking Cessation:**

Lena, a 28-year-old woman, had been smoking for over 10 years. She had tried quitting multiple times but always relapsed due to intense cravings and stress. After learning about EFT, Lena began using the technique to address both the physical cravings and the emotional triggers that led to her smoking. Through tapping, she reduced the intensity of her cravings and worked through the emotional triggers such as stress, anxiety, and past trauma. After several weeks of EFT, Lena found that her cravings had significantly decreased, and she was able to quit smoking for good.

EFT offers a holistic and effective approach to combating addiction by addressing both the emotional and physical aspects of the condition. By using tapping techniques to release emotional pain, reduce cravings, and reframe negative beliefs, individuals can regain control over their addictive behaviors and build a foundation for lasting recovery. Whether overcoming substance abuse, gambling, or smoking, EFT provides a powerful tool for those seeking to break free from addiction and create a healthier, more fulfilling life. With the growing number of success stories, it's clear that EFT is a valuable addition to addiction treatment and recovery strategies.

EFT to manage cravings and withdrawal symptoms

Cravings and withdrawal symptoms are common hurdles for individuals attempting to break free from addiction, whether it's related to substances such as nicotine, alcohol, or drugs, or even behavioral habits like overeating or gambling. These symptoms, often accompanied by intense emotional and physical discomfort, can make the recovery process feel insurmountable. However, Emotional Freedom Technique (EFT) offers an effective method for managing cravings and easing withdrawal symptoms by addressing both the emotional and physiological aspects of addiction.

How EFT Helps Manage Cravings and Withdrawal Symptoms

Cravings and withdrawal symptoms are not simply a result of the body's physical dependence on a substance; they are deeply linked to the mind's emotional responses and mental associations with that substance or behavior. In many cases, cravings are triggered by specific emotional states or stressful situations, such as feeling anxious, sad, or overwhelmed. EFT works by tapping on acupressure points on the body while focusing on the emotional or physical sensations associated with cravings or withdrawal, helping to neutralize the intensity of these urges and make them more manageable.

Here's how EFT helps with cravings and withdrawal symptoms:

1. **Emotional Regulation and Stress Relief:** One of the main reasons cravings and withdrawal symptoms arise is because of the body's heightened emotional response. EFT helps regulate the body's energy system, allowing the individual to calm the nervous system and release the emotional charge attached to cravings. For example, someone trying to quit smoking might feel an overwhelming urge to light up when they're stressed or anxious. By tapping while focusing on the specific emotion, the body's energy pathways are balanced, reducing the emotional intensity of the craving and providing relief.
2. **Releasing Emotional Triggers:** Cravings are often tied to specific emotional triggers, such as boredom, stress, or loneliness. These emotional triggers create an automatic mental and physical association with the substance or behavior in question. When an individual experiences these emotions, the brain prompts the urge to use the substance or engage in the addictive behavior. EFT works by identifying and addressing these emotional triggers directly. By tapping through

meridian points while focusing on the emotional experience, individuals can reduce the emotional charge and interrupt the cycle of cravings.

3. **Reducing Physical Withdrawal Symptoms:** Withdrawal symptoms can range from mild discomfort to severe physical reactions, such as headaches, fatigue, or nausea. EFT can help ease the physical symptoms by tapping on the body's acupressure points, which in turn may help release the body's tension and stress associated with withdrawal. For instance, someone withdrawing from caffeine may experience headaches. EFT can help ease this discomfort by focusing on the sensation of pain and tapping to release it, leading to a reduction in the intensity of the symptoms.

4. **Changing the Thought Patterns:** Cravings often come with intrusive thoughts or beliefs about the substance or behavior, such as "I can't function without this," or "I'll never be able to quit." These beliefs reinforce the addiction cycle and make cravings harder to resist. EFT helps change these thought patterns by tapping while focusing on the negative beliefs and replacing them with more empowering affirmations. For example, someone trying to quit drinking might tap while repeating, "Even though I feel I need alcohol to relax, I choose to feel calm and at peace without it." This shift in mindset reduces the psychological grip that the addiction has on the person.

5. **Creating New Associations:** Over time, individuals create strong mental associations between certain behaviors or situations and their addiction. For example, someone might always reach for a cigarette when they're driving or drink alcohol when they're socializing. EFT can help break these associations by targeting the emotional components attached to these triggers. By tapping on the specific memories or scenarios that lead to cravings, the person can change the emotional response and replace it with healthier alternatives, such as taking deep breaths or drinking water instead.

EFT Techniques to Manage Cravings and Withdrawal

Several EFT techniques are particularly helpful in managing cravings and withdrawal symptoms:

1. **Craving Reduction Technique:** This technique focuses directly on reducing the intensity of cravings. The individual taps while identifying the craving, such as, "Even though I feel this strong urge to smoke/drink/eat, I choose to release this craving now." As they tap through the meridian points, they focus on the specific sensations in the body that arise when they experience the craving, allowing these physical feelings to diminish. This technique helps reduce the emotional and physical intensity of the craving, making it easier to resist.

2. **The Emotional Root Technique:** Addiction often has deep emotional roots, such as trauma, stress, or negative beliefs that contribute to the cravings and withdrawal experience. By tapping on the emotional triggers behind the addiction—whether

they are past memories or current stressors—this technique helps to neutralize the emotional charge associated with them. For example, someone withdrawing from sugar may tap while focusing on the feelings of comfort they associate with eating sweets, helping to release that emotional connection.

3. **Physical Symptom Relief Technique:** This technique is used when dealing with physical withdrawal symptoms, such as headaches, nausea, or fatigue. The individual taps while focusing on the physical sensations, such as "Even though I have this headache, I choose to feel better and at ease." This technique can help to reduce the severity of physical symptoms and ease the body's response to withdrawal.

4. **The Reframing Technique:** Cravings and withdrawal are often fueled by negative thought patterns. The reframing technique involves tapping while focusing on these limiting beliefs or unhelpful thoughts. For example, a person who feels they are "powerless" in the face of their cravings might tap while repeating, "Even though I feel powerless, I choose to believe in my strength and ability to resist this urge." This technique helps shift the individual's mindset from one of helplessness to empowerment.

5. **Future Pacing:** Once cravings and withdrawal symptoms have been reduced, EFT can be used to visualize a future free from addiction. By tapping while imagining oneself successfully navigating situations without resorting to the addictive behavior, the individual can strengthen their belief in their ability to stay sober or refrain from the behavior. This technique also helps to establish new, healthier habits, reinforcing the commitment to a life without addiction.

Real-World Applications of EFT in Managing Cravings and Withdrawal

EFT has proven to be effective for managing cravings and withdrawal symptoms across a wide range of addictions. Here are a couple of examples:

1. **Managing Caffeine Withdrawal:**

Sarah, a 35-year-old woman, was a heavy coffee drinker who decided to quit caffeine. She experienced headaches, irritability, and fatigue as she withdrew from caffeine, making it difficult to stick to her goal. After learning EFT, Sarah began using it to manage her withdrawal symptoms. Each time she felt a headache or irritability, she would tap on the meridian points while focusing on the physical sensation, saying, "Even though I have this headache, I choose to relax and feel better." Over time, her symptoms diminished, and she was able to quit caffeine with much less discomfort.

2. **Overcoming Sugar Cravings:**

Tom, a 40-year-old man, had a sugar addiction that led to weight gain and poor health. He struggled with intense cravings, especially in the late afternoon, and found it hard to resist sugary snacks. Tom began using EFT to address his sugar cravings. Each time he felt the urge to indulge, he would tap on the craving while repeating, "Even though I want sugar, I choose to feel satisfied with healthy food." By focusing on the craving and tapping through the points, Tom was able to significantly reduce the intensity of his cravings and eventually break his addiction to sugar.

EFT offers a powerful tool for managing cravings and withdrawal symptoms, addressing both the emotional and physical aspects of addiction recovery. By tapping on specific acupressure points while focusing on cravings, negative beliefs, and emotional triggers, individuals can reduce the intensity of their urges and ease the discomfort of withdrawal. Whether someone is quitting smoking, alcohol, or other addictive behaviors, EFT can provide lasting relief and support in overcoming addiction. Through consistent practice, EFT helps individuals regain control, break free from unhealthy cycles, and build healthier habits for a balanced, addiction-free life.

Personal experience and stories

Personal experiences with Emotional Freedom Technique (EFT) highlight its transformative power in addressing a wide range of emotional, psychological, and physical challenges. Many individuals who have used EFT share stories of profound shifts in their lives, from overcoming long-standing anxiety and trauma to breaking free from addictive behaviors. These real-life accounts demonstrate how tapping on acupressure points while focusing on specific issues can bring about emotional healing and offer a sense of empowerment. Below are some powerful personal experiences that illustrate the effectiveness of EFT.

Overcoming Anxiety and Panic Attacks

Jennifer, a 34-year-old woman, had struggled with anxiety and panic attacks for most of her adult life. After years of therapy and medication, she still found herself overwhelmed by anxiety, particularly in social situations. She decided to try EFT after hearing about its ability to reduce emotional stress and anxiety. During her first session, Jennifer tapped while focusing on her fear of social interactions, repeating phrases such as, "Even though I am scared and anxious, I choose to feel calm and confident."

Within a few sessions, she noticed a significant reduction in her anxiety levels. Jennifer no longer experienced the same intense panic attacks when entering crowded spaces, and she began to feel more at ease in social settings. Over time, the emotional charge associated with her fear lessened, allowing her to manage situations that once felt overwhelming. Jennifer attributes her newfound peace and self-confidence to EFT, stating, "It's like a weight has been lifted off my shoulders. EFT has given me the tools to handle my emotions instead of feeling controlled by them."

Breaking Free from Addiction

Tom, a 40-year-old man, had been battling a gambling addiction for years. His addiction had led to financial instability and strained relationships, and he had tried numerous methods to quit, from counseling to self-help programs, with little success. Tom first heard about EFT through a friend who had used it to overcome smoking. Skeptical but desperate, he decided to give it a try.

During his initial EFT sessions, Tom focused on the emotional triggers that drove his need to gamble—feelings of boredom, stress, and a desire to escape from his everyday struggles. While tapping on the acupressure points, he would repeat affirmations such as, "Even though I feel the urge to gamble, I choose to let go of this addiction." Over the course of several weeks, Tom noticed a significant reduction in his cravings. He was no longer consumed by the desire to gamble, and he began to feel more in control of his decisions.

Tom's story is one of gradual recovery. While EFT didn't immediately solve all of his problems, it provided him with a tool to address the emotional root causes of his addiction, allowing him to resist the urge to gamble. Today, Tom is living a debt-free life, with healthier coping mechanisms and a renewed sense of hope. He credits EFT for giving him the emotional strength to face his addiction without feeling helpless.

Healing from Trauma

Sophie, a 28-year-old woman, had experienced a traumatic event in her teenage years that left her with deep emotional scars. Despite years of therapy, she continued to suffer from flashbacks, nightmares, and a persistent feeling of unease. After learning about EFT through an online support group, Sophie decided to try tapping to address her trauma.

Sophie's first experience with EFT was emotional. She tapped while focusing on the specific memories related to her trauma, repeating statements like, "Even though I feel scared and hurt because of what happened, I choose to heal and release this pain." The tapping process allowed Sophie to revisit the trauma in a way that felt safe, enabling her to process emotions she had long suppressed.

As Sophie continued to use EFT, the intensity of her flashbacks and nightmares gradually diminished. She found that tapping helped her stay grounded and calm when memories resurfaced. EFT didn't erase the trauma, but it allowed Sophie to process it in a healthier way, giving her a sense of emotional freedom that she hadn't experienced in years. "I feel lighter and more in control," she said. "EFT helped me reclaim my life from the shadows of the past."

Managing Chronic Pain

Michael, a 50-year-old man, had suffered from chronic back pain for several years. Despite seeing numerous specialists and trying various treatments, the pain persisted, impacting his quality of life. He learned about EFT from a colleague and was intrigued by its potential to address not just emotional issues, but physical ailments as well.

Michael began using EFT to target the pain in his back. As he tapped on the acupressure points, he focused on the sensation of discomfort, repeating phrases like, "Even though I have this pain in my back, I choose to release the tension and allow my body to heal." To his surprise, after just a few sessions, Michael noticed a decrease in the intensity of the pain. While it wasn't completely gone, he found that the pain was more manageable, and he could go about his day without feeling as restricted.

EFT gave Michael a new sense of control over his body. By tapping on the emotional and physical aspects of his pain, he was able to reduce its impact on his life. Michael now uses EFT as part of his regular wellness routine, often tapping to relieve tension or stress that may contribute to flare-ups. "EFT has been a game-changer," he shared. "It doesn't cure everything, but it helps me manage my pain in a way I never thought possible."

Overcoming Self-Doubt and Building Confidence

Rachel, a 42-year-old woman, struggled with deep-seated feelings of inadequacy and self-doubt. These feelings had held her back in both her personal and professional life. Rachel felt stuck in a cycle of negative thinking and believed she wasn't capable of achieving her goals. After hearing about EFT from a friend, she decided to try it in the hope that it would help her overcome her limiting beliefs.

During her EFT sessions, Rachel focused on the core beliefs that had been holding her back, such as, "I am not good enough," and "I will never succeed." She tapped while repeating positive affirmations such as, "Even though I feel like I'm not enough, I choose to accept myself as I am." Over time, Rachel began to notice a shift in her mindset. She felt more confident and began to take steps toward her goals without being paralyzed by fear of failure.

One year after starting EFT, Rachel landed a promotion at work and began pursuing a new career path she had always dreamed of. Reflecting on her progress, Rachel said, "EFT helped me break free from the mental blocks I had built for myself. It taught me to trust in my abilities and stop letting my fears control me."

These personal stories provide a glimpse into the transformative power of EFT in a variety of contexts, from overcoming addiction to managing pain, trauma, and self-doubt. While each person's experience with EFT is unique, a common thread runs through these accounts: EFT empowers individuals to address the emotional and psychological roots of their challenges, offering a tool for healing, growth, and self-empowerment. As these real-life examples show, EFT is not just a quick fix, but a tool for lasting change, helping individuals unlock their potential and reclaim control over their lives. Whether dealing with emotional distress, physical pain, or limiting beliefs, EFT offers a path to healing that is both accessible and deeply transformative.

Emotional Freedom for Kids

Children face a unique set of emotional challenges as they grow, including feelings of fear, anxiety, frustration, and sadness. Whether it's dealing with the stress of school, difficulty with social interactions, or experiencing the emotional ups and downs of childhood, kids often struggle to manage their emotions effectively. The Emotional Freedom Technique (EFT) offers a simple, effective tool to help children process and regulate their emotions in a healthy way. By tapping on acupressure points while focusing on specific issues, EFT allows kids to release emotional blockages, reduce stress, and cultivate emotional resilience.

How EFT Benefits Children

EFT taps into the body's energy system, using light fingertip pressure on specific acupressure points along the meridians to help balance energy and reduce emotional distress. Unlike traditional therapies that require verbal expression and analysis, EFT works through physical sensations and feelings, making it accessible and easy for children to understand and use. Children do not need to fully understand the psychological aspects of their emotions for EFT to be effective—what's most important is their ability to focus on how they feel in the moment.

For example, if a child feels anxious before a school test, EFT helps them focus on the anxiety they are experiencing. By tapping on the meridian points while saying affirmations like, "Even though I feel nervous about the test, I choose to be calm and confident," the child can release the intensity of their anxiety, helping them feel more in control of their emotions. This is particularly helpful for kids who struggle with verbalizing their feelings or have difficulty understanding the source of their emotions.

Managing Common Childhood Issues with EFT

1. Anxiety and Fear: Many children experience anxiety, whether it's due to separation from parents, fear of the dark, or stress about school. By addressing the root cause of these emotions, EFT can help reduce anxiety and fear. For example, a child who is afraid of going to the dentist might tap while focusing on their fear, repeating statements like, "Even though I am scared, I choose to feel safe and calm."

2. Anger and Frustration: Anger is a natural emotion, but when left unaddressed, it can lead to tantrums and other behavioral issues. EFT helps children process and release anger in a safe and controlled way. For instance, a child who is upset about losing a game might tap while focusing on their frustration, saying, "Even though I feel angry because I lost, I choose to feel calm and happy." This allows the child to release the emotional charge and regain control of their behavior.

3. Grief and Loss: Children may struggle with grief when they experience a loss, such as the death of a pet or a family member. EFT provides a gentle way for them to process the sadness and find emotional balance. By tapping while acknowledging their sadness, children can release pent-up emotions and start to heal. Statements like, "Even though I miss my pet, I choose to feel at peace" can help them process their grief without feeling overwhelmed.

4. Sleep Issues: Difficulty falling asleep is common among children, often due to anxiety, fear, or overactive minds. EFT can help children calm their nervous system and relax before bedtime. By tapping on points while focusing on relaxation and comfort, children can release any underlying stress that might be preventing them from falling asleep. Affirmations like, "Even though I feel restless, I choose to feel peaceful and relaxed" can help promote a calm and restful night's sleep.

5. School Stress: School-related stress is another common issue for children, from pressure to perform academically to navigating friendships. EFT can help children manage these stresses by addressing the emotional responses tied to their experiences. Whether it's dealing with test anxiety, worries about fitting in, or frustration with homework, EFT allows children to release negative emotions and approach their challenges with a clearer mind. Tapping while repeating affirmations like, "Even though I feel stressed about school, I choose to feel confident and capable" can boost a child's emotional resilience and help them face school with a positive mindset.

How to Introduce EFT to Children

Introducing EFT to children requires a gentle, playful approach that makes the technique engaging and accessible. Here are some tips for parents and caregivers looking to use EFT with children:

1. Make It Fun: Children respond well to playful activities, so frame EFT as a fun and interactive game. Use simple language and make tapping feel like a positive, enjoyable experience. You can even create a character or story around tapping to keep the child engaged. For example, you might tell a story about a superhero who uses tapping to stay calm in difficult situations.

2. Use Kid-Friendly Language: Keep the language simple and easy to understand. Instead of talking about energy systems and meridians, focus on how tapping helps children feel better. Use phrases that resonate with children, such as, "Tapping helps you feel stronger" or "This will help you feel calmer and happier."

3. Tap Along with the Child: Children are more likely to engage with EFT if they see you using it as well. Tap alongside the child while guiding them through the process, so they feel supported and confident in using the technique. Lead by example and show them that tapping is a tool they can use whenever they need help with their emotions.

4. Focus on Specific Issues: When teaching EFT to children, focus on a specific emotion or issue they are dealing with. Ask them to think about the feeling or situation that is bothering them, and guide them through the tapping process. Help them identify the emotions they are experiencing, such as fear, frustration, or sadness, and tap on those feelings until they feel better.

5. Keep Sessions Short: Children's attention spans are shorter than adults', so it's important to keep EFT sessions brief and focused. A typical EFT session for a child may only last a few minutes, but even a short session can be incredibly effective in helping them release intense emotions and regain a sense of calm.

Success Stories of EFT for Children

1. Overcoming Fear of the Dark: One young boy named Max had a persistent fear of the dark that made bedtime a nightly challenge. His mother introduced him to EFT, and together they tapped while focusing on his fear. Max repeated affirmations such as, "Even though I am scared of the dark, I choose to feel safe and relaxed." After just a few sessions, Max's fear of the dark lessened significantly, and he was able to sleep through the night without needing a nightlight.

2. Reducing School Anxiety: Emily, a 9-year-old girl, struggled with school anxiety, particularly before tests and presentations. Her mother used EFT to help her process these anxious feelings. Emily tapped while focusing on her fear of failing, saying, "Even though I'm worried about the test, I choose to feel calm and confident." Over time, Emily's anxiety decreased, and she found it easier to approach school with a positive mindset. By using EFT regularly, Emily learned to manage her school-related stress in a healthier way.

3. Coping with Loss: Sophie, a 6-year-old girl, was deeply affected by the death of her pet hamster. Her parents used EFT to help Sophie process her grief, tapping on the sadness while repeating phrases like, "Even though I miss my hamster, I choose to feel peaceful and happy." Sophie's emotional healing was supported by the tapping process, and over the next few weeks, her grief softened, and she was able to remember her pet fondly without feeling overwhelmed by sadness.

EFT is a powerful tool that can support children in managing their emotions, reducing stress, and cultivating emotional resilience. By incorporating tapping into daily routines, children can learn to process and release negative emotions, improve their self-regulation, and build coping skills that will serve them throughout their lives. Whether it's easing anxiety before a school test, calming anger after a frustrating situation, or helping a child cope with grief, EFT offers a gentle, non-invasive way to support emotional well-being. With its simple and effective approach, EFT empowers children to navigate their emotional worlds with greater ease and confidence.

EFT for different age groups

Emotional Freedom Technique (EFT) is a versatile tool that can be used across different age groups, offering tailored support to individuals at various stages of life. Its ability to address emotional, mental, and physical issues makes it a valuable tool for people of all ages, from young children to the elderly. By tapping on acupressure points while focusing on specific emotional challenges, EFT helps individuals release negative emotions, reduce stress, and regain emotional balance. Below is an exploration of how EFT can benefit different age groups, highlighting how the technique can be adapted to meet the unique needs of each stage of life.

EFT for Children

Children are naturally emotional and sensitive to their environments, which means they often experience strong feelings like anxiety, anger, and sadness. However, they may lack the emotional tools to effectively manage these feelings. EFT can help children process their emotions in a simple and effective way by using tapping to release emotional blockages.

For younger children, the process is typically very hands-on and playful. Parents can guide them through tapping sessions by making it fun and engaging. For example, a child dealing with fear of the dark can tap on the acupressure points while repeating phrases like, "Even though I am scared of the dark, I choose to feel calm and safe." The simplicity of EFT makes it particularly effective for kids, as they can focus on how they feel and the tapping itself without needing to fully understand complex psychological concepts. Children as young as three or four can start practicing EFT, especially with adult guidance.

EFT helps children manage common emotional challenges such as:

- **Anxiety** (e.g., fear of the dark, separation anxiety, test anxiety)
- **Anger and frustration** (e.g., tantrums, sibling rivalry)
- **Grief and loss** (e.g., death of a pet, moving to a new home)
- **Behavioral issues** (e.g., self-control difficulties, lack of focus)
- **School stress** (e.g., performance anxiety, peer pressure)

EFT for Teenagers

Adolescence is a time of immense change, both physically and emotionally. Teenagers often face heightened stress due to academic pressures, social challenges, and identity formation. These changes can lead to feelings of self-doubt, anxiety, and emotional overwhelm. EFT provides a simple yet powerful way for teenagers to address these emotions and develop greater emotional resilience.

Unlike younger children, teenagers can understand and articulate their emotions more clearly, so the focus during EFT sessions can be more reflective and self-aware. A teen dealing with test anxiety, for example, can tap while focusing on the specific stress they feel about their exams, saying something like, "Even though I feel overwhelmed by this test, I choose to feel calm and confident."

EFT can help teenagers:

- **Manage academic pressure** (e.g., fear of failure, procrastination, study stress)
- **Improve self-esteem** (e.g., body image issues, self-criticism)
- **Reduce anxiety and panic attacks** (e.g., social anxiety, performance anxiety)
- **Navigate relationships** (e.g., peer pressure, family dynamics, romantic relationships)
- **Curb negative thoughts** (e.g., self-doubt, perfectionism, fear of judgment)

EFT is especially effective for teenagers because it offers a non-judgmental space for them to deal with complex emotions. The technique's simplicity and direct approach help them quickly gain emotional relief, empowering them to manage their feelings without the need for extensive therapy sessions.

EFT for Adults

Adults face a wide range of emotional challenges throughout their lives, including work-related stress, relationship difficulties, financial concerns, and unresolved past trauma. EFT can be particularly beneficial for adults, as it allows them to address both current stressors and deeply rooted emotional issues in a manageable and effective way.

For adults, EFT can be used to tackle a variety of issues, including:

- **Stress management** (e.g., work stress, time management, family responsibilities)
- **Anxiety and depression** (e.g., chronic stress, generalized anxiety disorder, panic attacks)
- **Trauma recovery** (e.g., past abuse, PTSD, emotional wounds)
- **Addiction and cravings** (e.g., smoking, overeating, alcohol dependence)
- **Physical pain** (e.g., chronic pain, headaches, back pain)
- **Self-worth and personal growth** (e.g., fear of failure, self-doubt, limiting beliefs)

Adults can use EFT for emotional regulation, gaining clarity on their emotions and releasing negative patterns that may have been limiting their progress. EFT allows individuals to address specific emotional challenges in real-time, offering an immediate sense of relief. Many adults find that tapping becomes a valuable self-care tool that can be used whenever they feel overwhelmed, stressed, or emotionally drained.

EFT for Older Adults and Seniors

As individuals age, they may face a variety of physical, emotional, and mental challenges. For older adults, EFT can help manage the emotional difficulties that arise due to aging, such as the loss of loved ones, health issues, or feelings of loneliness. Additionally, seniors may experience grief, anxiety, or fear related to their health, loss of independence, or end-of-life concerns. EFT provides a way for seniors to address these feelings and regain a sense of emotional peace.

Seniors may benefit from EFT in the following ways:

- **Managing grief and loss** (e.g., death of a spouse, friends, or pets)
- **Alleviating physical pain** (e.g., arthritis, joint pain, chronic conditions)
- **Dealing with loneliness or isolation** (e.g., separation from family, living alone)
- **Reducing anxiety and depression** (e.g., fear of aging, medical concerns, changes in lifestyle)
- **Improving sleep** (e.g., insomnia, sleep disturbances related to stress)

Because EFT involves tapping on acupressure points, it can be a gentle practice for older adults, and it can be done at a slow pace that suits their physical and emotional needs. Many seniors find that EFT not only helps them with emotional well-being but also enhances their physical health by addressing the mind-body connection.

The Flexibility of EFT Across Age Groups

One of the greatest strengths of EFT is its adaptability across all age groups. It's a technique that can be tailored to the specific needs of individuals based on their age, developmental stage, and emotional challenges. For children and teenagers, EFT can be used to process immediate emotional upsets, fears, or stressors. For adults, it serves as a tool for addressing more complex emotional issues, from past trauma to ongoing relationship struggles. For seniors, EFT offers a gentle yet powerful way to manage the emotional and physical changes that come with aging.

EFT is particularly effective because it focuses on both the emotional and physical aspects of stress, making it a holistic approach to emotional healing. It's a self-empowerment tool that allows individuals to take control of their emotional well-being, no matter their age. Whether it's a young child learning how to calm themselves, a teenager gaining confidence, or an adult processing years of trauma, EFT provides a pathway to emotional freedom at any stage of life.

In conclusion, Emotional Freedom Technique is a valuable tool for people of all ages. Whether helping children manage anxiety or guiding seniors through grief, EFT offers a versatile approach to emotional healing. Its simplicity, accessibility, and effectiveness make it an invaluable resource for anyone looking to improve their emotional health, no matter their age or life experience.

Techniques to teach children EFT

Teaching children the Emotional Freedom Technique (EFT) can be a powerful tool for helping them manage their emotions, alleviate stress, and improve emotional regulation. EFT involves tapping on specific acupressure points on the body while focusing on a particular issue, feeling, or stressor. This technique helps release emotional blockages and promotes emotional healing. When teaching EFT to children, it's important to make the process simple, fun, and engaging, so they can easily understand and benefit from it. Here are several strategies and techniques to help children learn EFT in a way that resonates with them.

1. Make It Playful and Fun

Children respond best to activities that are engaging and enjoyable. To teach EFT, consider turning the process into a fun game or story. Use imaginative language to keep their attention and make tapping feel like an enjoyable activity. For example, you can create a story around the tapping process, like turning the acupressure points into superheroes that help fight off "bad feelings" or "negative energy."

A fun idea might be to explain the tapping points as places on their body where they can send "positive energy" to feel better. You could say, "This spot here on the top of your head is like a magic button that helps you feel calm." By using playful language, you can make the process of tapping exciting and relatable for children.

2. Use Simple Language

When explaining EFT to children, it's important to use clear and simple language that they can easily understand. Avoid overwhelming them with technical terms, and instead focus on how tapping can help them feel better. For example, instead of talking about "meridians" or "energy blocks," explain that tapping helps them feel calm, confident, or brave when they're upset.

You might say, "Tapping helps us feel less worried, less sad, or less angry. It's like giving our feelings a hug." This keeps the focus on the emotional benefits of tapping, which will be easier for a child to grasp.

3. Start with a Simple Issue

For young children, it's best to start with a simple issue that they can easily relate to, such as fear of the dark, anxiety about school, or frustration over a toy. Help the child identify a feeling they want to address, then guide them through the tapping process. For example, if the child is feeling nervous about going to school, you can have them say, "Even though I feel nervous about school, I choose to feel brave."

Starting with a specific, small issue will make the experience more manageable for the child and help them feel a sense of accomplishment once they see that tapping has made a difference.

4. Tap Along with Them

Children often feel more comfortable learning new techniques when they see adults doing it with them. Tap alongside your child while guiding them through the process, so they feel supported and not alone. You can model the tapping process and say the affirmations aloud for them to follow, providing a sense of reassurance and encouragement.

For example, you can tap on the points while saying, "Even though I'm feeling nervous, I choose to feel calm," and encourage your child to repeat after you. This shows them that EFT is something they can do with help and that it's okay to be vulnerable and open about their feelings.

5. Use Affirmations that Resonate with Children

Affirmations play a key role in EFT because they help children reframe negative thoughts and focus on positive outcomes. When working with children, it's important to use affirmations that are easy for them to say and that make sense in their world.

For example, a child who is afraid of the dark might say, "Even though I'm scared of the dark, I choose to feel safe." For a child who is upset about a conflict with a friend, you could use, "Even though I feel angry, I choose to feel calm and happy again." Make sure the language is positive and empowering, helping the child focus on the emotion they want to feel rather than the negative one they want to release.

6. Keep Sessions Short and Simple

Children have shorter attention spans, so it's important to keep EFT sessions brief and focused. A tapping session for a child might only take 5-10 minutes, especially in the beginning. It's also helpful to focus on just one issue at a time, so the child doesn't feel overwhelmed by trying to tackle multiple emotions or concerns in one session.

If the child enjoys the process, they may ask to do more tapping, but it's important to respect their attention span and emotional readiness. Consistency is key, so regular, shorter sessions are better than lengthy ones that may cause frustration or disengagement.

7. Use Visuals and Stories

Children are often visual learners, so using pictures or stories to explain EFT can be an effective method. For example, you could draw a simple picture of a child tapping on different points or use a child-friendly chart that shows where the tapping points are located.

You can also use stories that show how tapping helps. Create a narrative about a character who uses tapping to solve their emotional problems. This could be a fictional story where a superhero uses tapping to defeat feelings of fear or a fairy who taps to feel confident before her performance. Visuals and storytelling will help make the process feel more familiar and engaging to children.

8. Incorporate Breathing Techniques

EFT and deep breathing go hand-in-hand in promoting relaxation and reducing emotional intensity. When teaching children EFT, you can incorporate deep breathing exercises into the tapping process to help them calm down and focus. Before beginning the tapping sequence, guide them through a few deep breaths, saying, "Let's take a deep breath in and let it out slowly. This will help us feel relaxed."

By combining tapping with deep breathing, children can learn how to soothe their nervous system and regulate their emotions effectively.

9. Use Physical Activities to Reinforce Tapping

Children are naturally active, and sometimes sitting still for tapping can feel challenging for them. If this is the case, allow the child to move around while tapping. They can stand, jump, or tap while walking to release extra energy. You can even use creative movement to make the tapping more interactive, such as having them pretend to be a superhero who uses tapping to stay strong and brave.

If the child is having trouble focusing or staying still, incorporate dancing or jumping into the tapping routine to keep their energy engaged. Movement can make the practice feel more enjoyable and can help children stay focused on the task.

10. Encourage Regular Use of EFT

One of the best ways to help children master EFT is to encourage them to use it regularly. Once they are familiar with the tapping process, encourage them to use it on their own when they are feeling anxious, upset, or stressed. Reinforce the idea that tapping is a tool they can use anytime they need to feel better.

Remind them that it's okay to tap when they are feeling angry, sad, or nervous, and that EFT is a way to help them regain control of their emotions. The more frequently children use EFT, the more it becomes a natural tool for emotional self-regulation.

Teaching EFT to children is an effective way to help them manage their emotions and navigate the challenges they face in daily life. By making the process fun, simple, and interactive, children can quickly learn how to tap into their emotional resilience. Whether they're managing school anxiety, fear of the dark, or frustration with friends, EFT offers children a powerful tool for self-soothing and emotional healing. With regular practice and support, children can develop emotional intelligence and confidence that will serve them throughout their lives.

Success stories from pediatric EFT

Emotional Freedom Technique (EFT) has been increasingly recognized for its effectiveness in helping children manage a variety of emotional and behavioral challenges. Through tapping on specific acupressure points while focusing on emotional issues, EFT helps children release emotional blockages and reduce stress, anxiety, and trauma. Over the years, numerous success stories have emerged from parents, caregivers, and therapists who have seen dramatic improvements in children's emotional health through EFT. Below are a few notable success stories demonstrating the power of this technique in pediatric care.

Overcoming Anxiety and Fear of the Dark

One of the most common issues parents seek help for is childhood anxiety, particularly fear of the dark. Many children experience intense fear at night, which can interfere with their ability to sleep and their overall sense of safety. In one case, a six-year-old girl named Sophie had an overwhelming fear of the dark, which began after watching a scary movie. Sophie would become distressed every evening when it was time to go to bed, refusing to enter her room and often having panic attacks.

Her mother, after learning about EFT, decided to try it as a solution. They started with Sophie identifying her fear and acknowledging the intensity of her feelings. Together, they tapped through the basic EFT points, repeating phrases like, "Even though I am scared of the dark, I choose to feel calm and safe." After a few sessions, Sophie reported feeling much more at ease at night, and her anxiety about the dark significantly diminished. Her mother said that Sophie was able to enter her room and go to bed without the usual tears and fear.

Within a few weeks of regular EFT sessions, Sophie's fear was completely gone, and she no longer had trouble sleeping. This success story highlights how EFT can be a gentle yet powerful way to address childhood fears and anxieties.

Managing School Anxiety

Another common issue children face is anxiety about school, whether due to social pressures, academic challenges, or separation anxiety. Liam, a 9-year-old boy, struggled with school-related anxiety. He would often experience stomach aches and cry before going to school, and he frequently asked his mother to let him stay home. The source of his anxiety was rooted in a fear of being judged by his peers and not doing well in his schoolwork.

After working with an EFT practitioner, Liam learned how to use tapping to address his fears. He tapped on the points while focusing on the feelings of fear and pressure that arose when he thought about school. He used affirmations such as, "Even though I'm scared I won't do well at school, I choose to feel confident and capable."

Over several sessions, Liam's anxiety significantly decreased. His stomach aches lessened, and he was able to go to school without feeling overwhelmed. His mother noted a marked change in his behavior—he became more confident and even started looking forward to school days. EFT helped Liam reframe his beliefs about school and build emotional resilience in the face of his fears.

Overcoming Anger and Behavioral Issues

Some children struggle with anger and behavioral issues, often as a result of frustration or difficulty managing their emotions. Jacob, an 8-year-old boy with a history of anger outbursts, was frequently acting out in school and at home. His parents were concerned about his temper, which seemed to escalate over time, especially when he was asked to do tasks he didn't enjoy, like homework.

Jacob's parents decided to introduce him to EFT. Initially, Jacob was skeptical about tapping and repeating affirmations, but once he understood that EFT was a way to feel better, he became more engaged. During sessions, Jacob tapped on the points while focusing on his feelings of frustration and anger, repeating phrases like, "Even though I'm angry, I choose to feel calm and in control."

After a few weeks of consistent tapping, Jacob's parents noticed a dramatic improvement in his behavior. He was less prone to anger outbursts, and his emotional regulation improved significantly. In school, he was able to focus better and respond to challenges with more patience. Jacob's parents were relieved to see him managing his emotions more effectively, and they continued using EFT as a tool for him to self-regulate his behavior.

Helping with Sleep Issues and Nightmares

Sleep problems are another area where EFT has proven to be effective for children. Ella, a 7-year-old girl, had been experiencing frequent nightmares for several months, which caused her to wake up distressed and unable to fall back asleep. Her parents tried various strategies, such as nightlights and calming bedtime routines, but nothing seemed to work.

After a recommendation from a friend, Ella's parents introduced EFT as a bedtime ritual. They tapped together on the points while focusing on the specific nightmares and feelings of fear. Ella would say, "Even though I'm scared of my nightmares, I choose to feel safe and calm when I sleep."

Within a few weeks of using EFT before bedtime, Ella began sleeping more soundly and reported fewer nightmares. She felt more relaxed and at ease when going to bed, and the frequency of nightmares decreased significantly. Her parents were impressed with how quickly EFT helped Ella, and they continued to use the technique as a tool for emotional self-regulation.

Supporting Children with ADHD

EFT has also shown promise in helping children with Attention Deficit Hyperactivity Disorder (ADHD). One young boy, Ethan, struggled with hyperactivity, impulsivity, and difficulty focusing in school. His parents had tried multiple strategies to help him manage his symptoms, but his behavior was still a challenge.

Ethan's therapist introduced EFT as part of his emotional regulation routine. Through tapping, Ethan learned to focus on his feelings of restlessness and frustration, using affirmations like, "Even though I feel like I can't sit still, I choose to feel calm and focused." Over time, his parents and teachers noticed improvements in his attention span and his ability to manage his impulses. Ethan's overall behavior became more balanced, and he was able to focus better in school and at home.

This case highlights how EFT can be used as a complementary tool for children with ADHD, helping them regulate their emotions and improve their focus and behavior.

These success stories illustrate the wide range of emotional challenges that EFT can address for children. Whether it's anxiety, fear, anger, sleep issues, or ADHD, EFT offers a gentle and non-invasive tool to help children manage their emotions and overcome behavioral challenges. By tapping on specific acupressure points while focusing on their feelings, children can gain emotional relief, build resilience, and develop healthy coping strategies for the future. The positive results seen in these stories demonstrate the transformative power of EFT in pediatric care and its potential as an effective tool for emotional healing and growth.

EFT in Relationship Management

Emotional Freedom Technique (EFT) is not only effective for individual emotional issues but also offers valuable tools for improving and managing relationships. Whether dealing with conflicts in romantic relationships, family dynamics, friendships, or workplace interactions, EFT helps individuals process and release emotional blockages that may be hindering communication, trust, and overall relationship health. By tapping on specific acupressure points while focusing on negative emotions or relationship-related issues, EFT can promote emotional healing and improve interactions with others.

Addressing Emotional Triggers in Relationships

In any relationship, certain events or behaviors can trigger strong emotional reactions. These triggers may stem from past experiences, unresolved issues, or deep-seated fears. For example, a partner might feel hurt or angry when their significant other forgets a special occasion or fails to communicate effectively. These emotional responses can sometimes lead to misunderstandings or conflicts.

EFT is an excellent tool for managing these emotional triggers. By tapping on the acupressure points while focusing on the specific trigger and repeating affirmations like, "Even though I feel hurt when this happens, I choose to feel calm and open," individuals can begin to release the intense emotional reactions associated with these triggers. This can help create a more balanced emotional response and open up healthier communication channels.

Healing Past Wounds and Resentments

In many relationships, unresolved past wounds and resentments can fester over time, leading to bitterness or ongoing conflicts. Old emotional baggage from past relationships or childhood experiences can carry over into current relationships, affecting how we interact with others. For instance, someone might have difficulty trusting their partner due to past betrayals or might react defensively due to childhood experiences of criticism or neglect.

EFT can be incredibly effective in helping individuals heal from these past emotional wounds. By tapping on the points while focusing on the pain or resentment, individuals can work through negative emotions tied to past experiences. With consistent tapping, they can gradually shift their mindset, allowing them to release old patterns and approach their relationships with greater understanding, empathy, and emotional balance.

Enhancing Communication and Reducing Conflict

Communication is a key factor in any healthy relationship, but emotional barriers can sometimes make it difficult to communicate openly and effectively. When individuals feel defensive, anxious, or misunderstood, they may struggle to express themselves clearly, which can lead to escalating conflicts. EFT can help reduce these emotional barriers by promoting emotional regulation and helping individuals stay calm in tense situations.

Before or during difficult conversations, individuals can use EFT to calm their nerves, clear their minds, and approach the discussion with greater clarity and openness. Tapping on the acupressure points while focusing on the issue at hand can help alleviate feelings of anxiety, anger, or frustration, creating space for more productive communication. A partner might tap and say, "Even though I feel frustrated right now, I choose to stay calm and listen to understand," which helps foster a more respectful and empathetic dialogue.

Building Trust and Emotional Intimacy

Trust is a foundational element in any relationship, but it can take time to build, especially if there have been past breaches of trust or emotional injuries. EFT can be a powerful tool in rebuilding trust and enhancing emotional intimacy. By helping individuals release the fear or anxiety tied to vulnerability, EFT can create an environment where partners feel safe to open up and share their feelings without judgment.

For example, if one partner has a history of being betrayed, they may feel hesitant to fully trust their current partner. By tapping on the negative emotions tied to this fear, they can release the emotional charge and open themselves up to the possibility of building a trusting connection. Affirmations like, "Even though I have been hurt in the past, I choose to trust and be vulnerable in this relationship," can be used during the tapping process to shift these limiting beliefs.

Improving Self-Awareness and Empathy

In relationships, self-awareness plays a key role in understanding how our emotions and behaviors impact others. EFT can enhance self-awareness by encouraging individuals to examine their feelings, beliefs, and responses to certain situations. Through tapping, individuals can gain deeper insight into their emotional triggers, patterns, and the underlying causes of their reactions.

As individuals become more aware of their emotional responses, they can develop greater empathy for their partner's experiences and emotions. EFT helps foster emotional intelligence by allowing individuals to recognize and release reactive patterns, leading to more compassionate and understanding relationships.

For instance, if one partner frequently reacts with anger when feeling criticized, tapping can help them identify and address the underlying fear or insecurity that triggers the anger. This increased self-awareness allows the partner to approach their reactions with more understanding and compassion, ultimately improving the relationship dynamic.

Managing Jealousy and Insecurity

Jealousy and insecurity are common emotional challenges that can create tension and instability in relationships. Whether it's jealousy of a partner's friendships, insecurities about personal appearance, or fear of abandonment, these emotions can undermine trust and intimacy.

EFT can help individuals address these feelings of jealousy and insecurity by focusing on the underlying fears and negative beliefs. For example, someone who feels insecure in their relationship may tap on the points while focusing on their fear of losing their partner, using affirmations like, "Even though I feel insecure, I choose to trust myself and my relationship." This practice can help shift the individual's mindset, reduce anxiety, and create a stronger sense of security within the relationship.

Strengthening Long-Term Relationships

EFT can be especially beneficial for couples who have been together for a long time and may be facing issues such as emotional distance, routine, or a lack of connection. As relationships mature, partners may experience a decline in emotional intimacy or face challenges in maintaining a strong connection.

By using EFT regularly, couples can work together to address any emotional blockages or unresolved issues that may arise over time. Tapping can help partners stay emotionally in tune with each other, prevent misunderstandings, and reinforce a sense of mutual respect and affection. For example, a couple experiencing a lack of intimacy might tap together, focusing on feelings of closeness, trust, and connection. With consistent use, EFT can help couples stay emotionally grounded and continue to nurture their bond.

EFT offers a wide array of benefits for relationship management, providing individuals with a tool to address emotional triggers, heal past wounds, enhance communication, and foster trust and intimacy. By tapping on specific acupressure points while focusing on relationship challenges, individuals can release negative emotions, improve self-

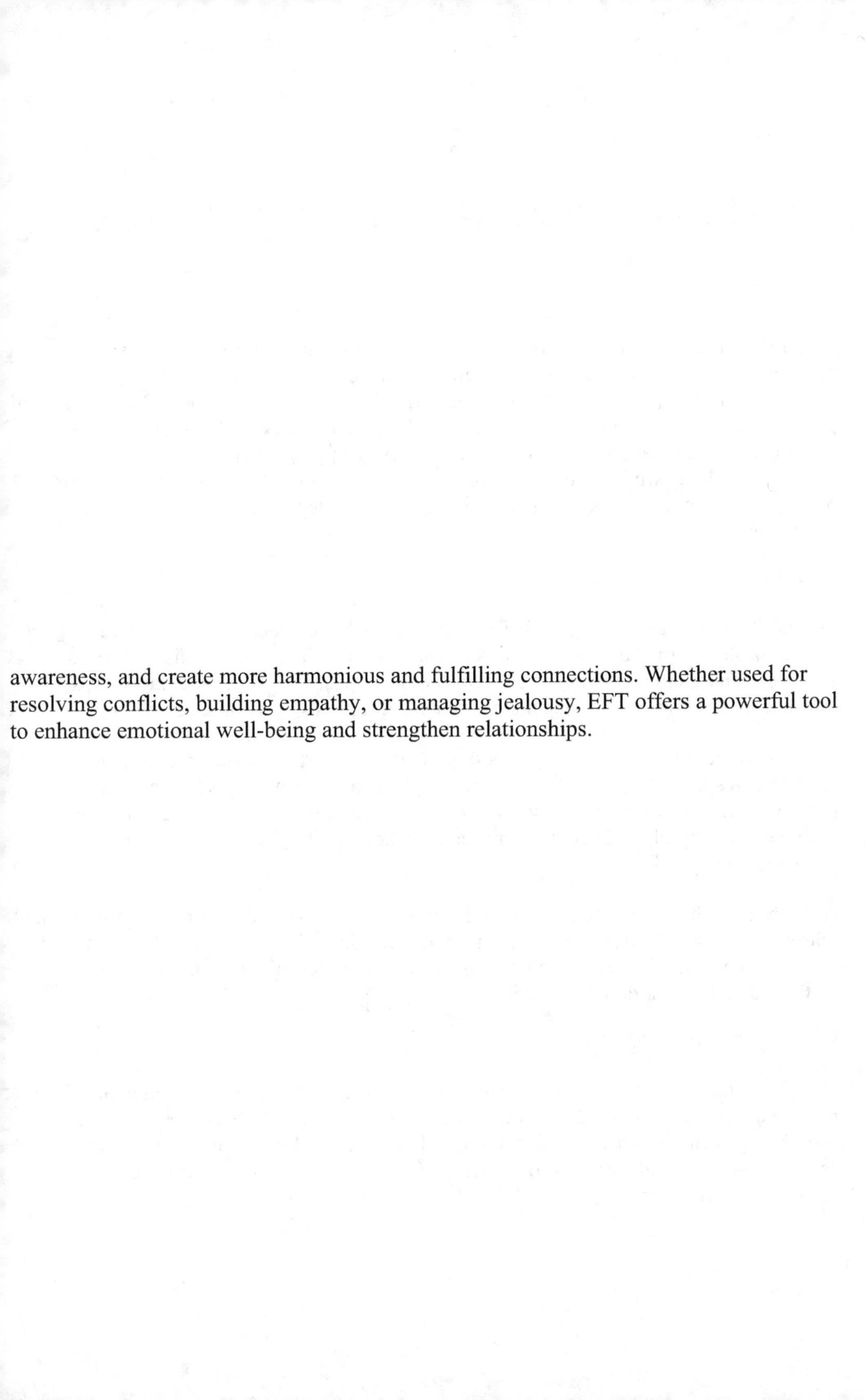

awareness, and create more harmonious and fulfilling connections. Whether used for resolving conflicts, building empathy, or managing jealousy, EFT offers a powerful tool to enhance emotional well-being and strengthen relationships.

How to use EFT in relationships

Emotional Freedom Technique (EFT) is a versatile tool that can be effectively used in relationships to address emotional triggers, reduce conflicts, and promote deeper understanding and intimacy. Whether you're dealing with miscommunication, unresolved past issues, or emotional challenges, EFT can help you process difficult emotions and foster healthier interactions. The technique involves tapping on specific acupressure points on the body while focusing on negative emotions or issues. This process helps release emotional blockages, regulate feelings, and create space for better emotional responses.

Identifying Emotional Triggers in Relationships

One of the first steps in using EFT within a relationship is identifying emotional triggers. In relationships, small actions or words can sometimes trigger strong, disproportionate reactions. These emotional triggers often stem from past experiences or unresolved issues, and they can lead to misunderstandings, arguments, or feelings of hurt.

To address these triggers with EFT, both partners can start by acknowledging the emotional response they're having. For example, if one partner feels hurt after a perceived criticism, they can focus on the specific emotional reaction and tap while saying something like, "Even though I feel hurt and upset by what was said, I choose to feel calm and open."

As both individuals tap through the points, they can process their emotional reactions and release the intense feelings tied to the trigger. Over time, this can reduce the emotional charge associated with specific situations, making it easier to communicate without getting caught in emotional reactivity.

Clearing Past Wounds and Resentments

Many relationship difficulties stem from past wounds or accumulated resentments. These may be old issues or misunderstandings that have never been fully addressed, often resurfacing during moments of stress or conflict. EFT can help clear these old emotional scars by allowing both partners to process the pain and release the negative energy that has built up over time.

To address past wounds, partners can tap on the specific emotional issues, using statements like, "Even though I'm still hurt by what happened in the past, I choose to release this pain and forgive." EFT helps bring awareness to these unresolved emotions, allowing both partners to let go of lingering resentment and create a more positive emotional foundation in their relationship.

Enhancing Communication and Reducing Conflict

Communication is key to any successful relationship, yet it can sometimes become challenging when emotions run high. When partners feel misunderstood, defensive, or emotionally charged, it can be difficult to communicate clearly and productively. EFT can be used to calm emotional reactions and create space for more open, honest communication.

Before or during a difficult conversation, both partners can use EFT to tap through any negative emotions they may be feeling. For example, if one partner is feeling anxious or defensive before a discussion, they can tap on the points while focusing on those feelings, saying things like, "Even though I feel nervous and defensive, I choose to stay calm and open to hearing my partner's perspective."

By reducing emotional intensity, EFT helps create a more neutral emotional state, allowing both individuals to engage in the conversation without being overwhelmed by fear, anger, or frustration. This can lead to a more productive, compassionate discussion, even on difficult topics.

Building Trust and Emotional Intimacy

Trust is the cornerstone of any healthy relationship, and EFT can be a powerful tool for rebuilding or strengthening trust. Whether trust has been damaged by past mistakes or external circumstances, EFT can help individuals process the emotions tied to fear, betrayal, or insecurity and rebuild a sense of emotional safety.

For example, if one partner is struggling with trust issues, they can use EFT to tap on feelings of fear or vulnerability. A statement like, "Even though I'm afraid of being hurt again, I choose to trust my partner and feel safe in this relationship," can help reduce the emotional charge around the fear and promote emotional healing. By tapping regularly on these emotions, partners can begin to feel more secure and open with each other, which is essential for deepening emotional intimacy.

Strengthening Empathy and Understanding

EFT can also be used to increase empathy and understanding between partners. Often, conflicts arise because each partner feels misunderstood or not fully heard. By tapping on emotional reactions and focusing on the feelings and perspectives of both individuals,

EFT helps create a shared emotional experience that promotes empathy and understanding.

When one partner is upset, the other can tap along with them while repeating phrases like, "Even though my partner is feeling hurt, I choose to listen with compassion and try to understand their feelings." This allows the other person to stay emotionally present and supportive rather than defensive or dismissive. With consistent use of EFT, both partners can cultivate greater emotional intelligence and empathy, which can transform the way they relate to one another.

Managing Jealousy, Insecurity, and Other Negative Emotions

Negative emotions like jealousy, insecurity, or fear of abandonment can create tension in relationships and undermine trust and closeness. These feelings often stem from deep-rooted fears or past experiences, but EFT can help process and release these emotions.

For example, if one partner feels jealous about their significant other's friendships or interactions with others, they can use EFT to tap on feelings of jealousy and insecurity. By saying, "Even though I feel jealous and afraid of losing my partner, I choose to release this fear and trust in our relationship," they can release the emotional charge and create space for more trust and security.

Regular tapping on these types of emotions can help both partners feel more confident and emotionally stable in the relationship, reducing the likelihood of misunderstandings or unnecessary conflict.

Using EFT Together as a Couple

In addition to using EFT individually, couples can also practice tapping together to address relationship challenges. This shared experience can be bonding and can help both individuals feel more aligned and connected. During a tapping session, both partners can focus on the same issue and tap through it together, which creates a sense of unity and mutual support.

For instance, if a couple is facing challenges with communication, they can tap together while focusing on the emotional barriers that hinder open dialogue. Tapping together allows both partners to release their emotions in real-time and move forward with greater understanding and compassion.

Using EFT in relationships can be a transformative tool for improving communication, reducing emotional reactivity, and fostering trust and intimacy. By tapping on acupressure points while focusing on specific relationship issues, both partners can process and release negative emotions, address past wounds, and strengthen their emotional connection. Whether dealing with jealousy, resentment, or miscommunication, EFT offers a gentle yet effective way to create healthier, more fulfilling relationships. By using EFT as a regular practice, couples can improve their emotional resilience and create a deeper sense of mutual understanding and respect.

Tools for conflict resolution

Conflict is an inevitable part of any relationship, but how it's handled can make all the difference between resolution and escalation. Emotional Freedom Technique (EFT) offers a set of tools that can significantly improve conflict resolution by addressing the emotional triggers that fuel disputes. Using tapping to balance the body's energy and shift negative emotions, EFT can help individuals and couples manage their reactions, communicate more effectively, and find common ground.

Identifying Emotional Triggers

One of the first steps in resolving conflict is identifying emotional triggers. Often, conflicts become heated not because of the issue at hand but due to underlying emotions, past experiences, or personal insecurities. When partners or individuals react with anger, frustration, or defensiveness, these emotional responses often stem from unresolved issues or deeply ingrained beliefs.

Using EFT, individuals can tap on specific acupressure points while focusing on the emotion they're feeling. By doing so, they release the intensity of the emotion and make space for clearer thinking and a more measured response. For example, someone might say while tapping, "Even though I feel triggered and angry when this happens, I choose to feel calm and listen with an open mind." This allows both individuals to address the emotional undercurrents of the conflict before it escalates.

Releasing Negative Emotions

In conflict situations, emotions can cloud judgment and make it difficult to see the other person's perspective. EFT helps individuals release the negative emotions that often fuel conflict, such as anger, resentment, fear, or sadness. By reducing the intensity of these emotions, both parties are better able to engage in a constructive dialogue.

During a conflict, one person might feel overwhelmed by their emotions, making it difficult to communicate effectively. Using EFT, they can tap on their emotional state, saying something like, "Even though I feel hurt and upset right now, I choose to release this emotion and approach this conversation with a calm heart." This simple technique can help both individuals regain emotional balance and prevent conflict from spiraling.

Improving Communication

Effective communication is essential for conflict resolution. However, during emotionally charged situations, it can be difficult to listen and respond without becoming defensive. EFT helps individuals manage their emotional responses, making it easier to engage in calm, respectful conversations.

One of the most powerful tools in EFT is its ability to create emotional regulation. When both partners tap during a conflict, they can lower emotional intensity and shift their focus toward resolving the issue rather than defending their position. For example, if a disagreement arises over a sensitive topic, both individuals can tap while focusing on their emotions, saying things like, "Even though we see this situation differently, I choose to listen with empathy and understanding." This sets the stage for open dialogue, where both parties can feel heard and respected.

Shifting Beliefs and Perspectives

Often, conflicts arise from different belief systems or perspectives, and it's easy to become entrenched in one's own viewpoint. EFT helps individuals shift their perspective by addressing the underlying emotional charge attached to their beliefs. For example, someone might be holding onto a belief that their partner doesn't care about their feelings, which causes defensiveness and tension when a disagreement arises.

By tapping on this belief, individuals can begin to release the negative emotions tied to it. A simple tapping statement could be, "Even though I feel like my partner doesn't care about my feelings, I choose to release this belief and open myself to understanding." By tapping through these negative beliefs, both parties can approach the conflict with a more open mind and greater empathy, reducing the likelihood of a prolonged disagreement.

Creating Space for Empathy and Understanding

Empathy is a key element in resolving conflicts, but it can be hard to achieve when emotions are running high. EFT can help individuals tap into their own emotional experience, allowing them to better empathize with the feelings of others. When both parties focus on their own emotional triggers during a conflict and tap to release the charge, they are more likely to understand each other's point of view.

For example, a person might feel misunderstood during a conflict, leading to frustration. By tapping on the feeling of being misunderstood, they release the emotional charge and can approach the conversation with an open heart. They may then be able to recognize their partner's emotional experience and engage more compassionately, saying something like, "I understand how you might feel upset, and I'm willing to listen and find a solution together." This creates a collaborative approach to resolving the issue, rather than a combative one.

Using EFT as a Couple

Couples can use EFT together during a conflict to help maintain emotional balance and prevent arguments from escalating. By tapping together while focusing on the same issue, both partners can address their emotional responses simultaneously, which can strengthen their emotional connection and promote cooperation.

For example, if a couple is arguing over household responsibilities, they can tap while focusing on their feelings about the situation. Statements like, "Even though I feel frustrated about this, I choose to stay calm and work together to find a solution," help both partners release tension and refocus on resolving the problem collaboratively. Regular tapping can also build emotional resilience over time, allowing couples to navigate future conflicts with greater ease.

Reaffirming Love and Commitment

During conflicts, it's easy to lose sight of the emotional connection that exists in the relationship. EFT can help reaffirm the love and commitment that partners have for one another, even when disagreements arise. Tapping together while focusing on feelings of love and appreciation can help couples reconnect emotionally and prevent conflicts from threatening the relationship.

For example, if a conflict has left both partners feeling distant, they can tap on statements like, "Even though we've had a disagreement, I choose to remember how much I love you and appreciate you." This helps shift the focus from the conflict to the underlying bond, reminding both individuals that their connection is stronger than any temporary disagreement.

Preventing Future Conflicts

EFT isn't only useful for resolving current conflicts—it can also help prevent future issues by addressing emotional triggers and underlying beliefs that may contribute to ongoing problems. Couples can use EFT regularly to maintain emotional balance and ensure that small issues don't snowball into larger, more damaging conflicts.

For example, a couple who frequently argues about finances can tap on their feelings around money, such as fear, stress, or insecurity, to reduce emotional tension before these issues arise. Tapping on these emotions regularly helps reduce the emotional charge around specific topics, allowing for more constructive discussions in the future.

EFT offers a range of tools for conflict resolution that focus on addressing the emotional components of disputes. By helping individuals and couples identify emotional triggers,

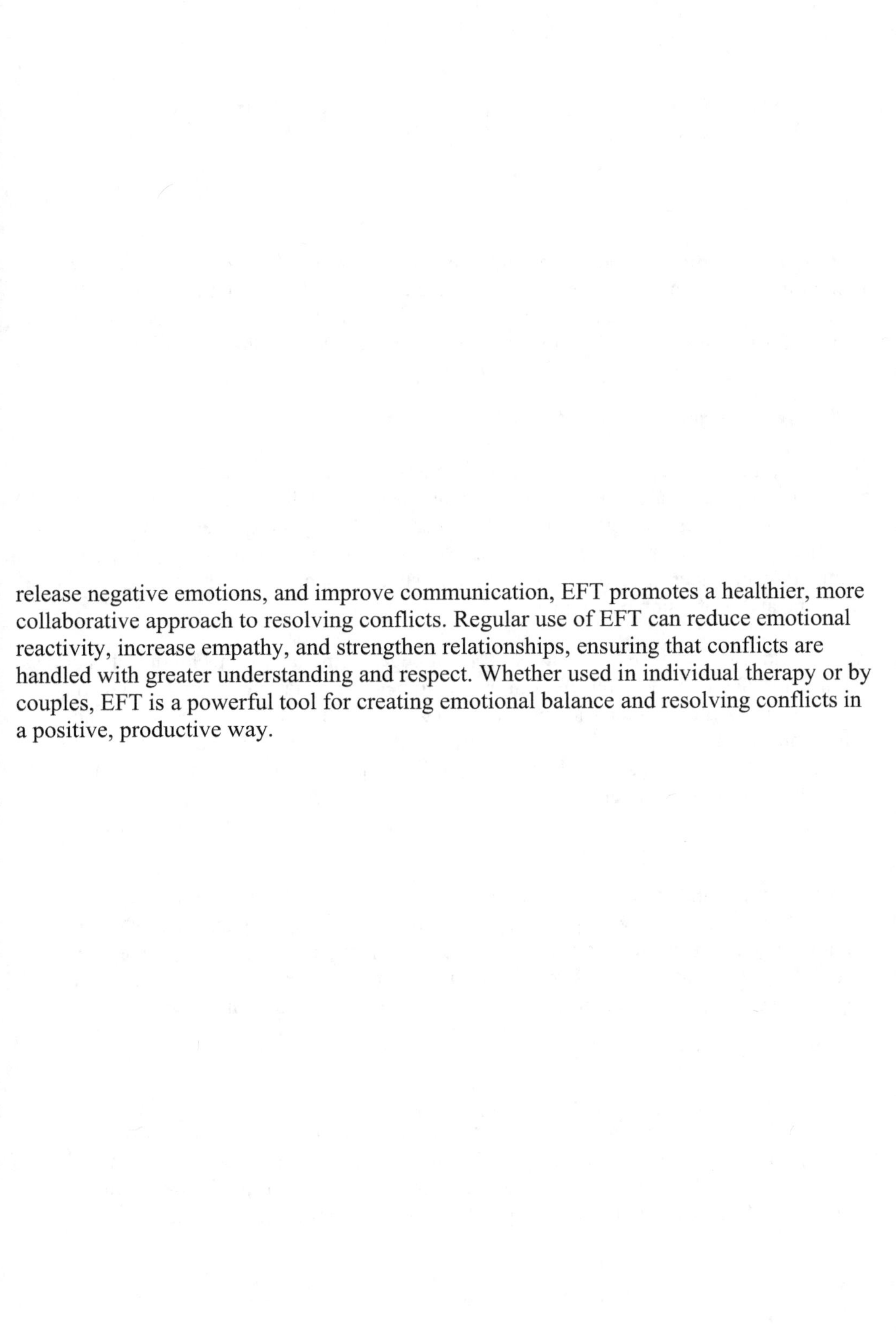

release negative emotions, and improve communication, EFT promotes a healthier, more collaborative approach to resolving conflicts. Regular use of EFT can reduce emotional reactivity, increase empathy, and strengthen relationships, ensuring that conflicts are handled with greater understanding and respect. Whether used in individual therapy or by couples, EFT is a powerful tool for creating emotional balance and resolving conflicts in a positive, productive way.

Case studies and practical advice

Case studies and practical advice provide invaluable insight into how Emotional Freedom Technique (EFT) can be used effectively to manage a variety of emotional issues, from stress and anxiety to trauma and relationship challenges. Real-life examples demonstrate the transformative power of tapping, and the guidance offered can help individuals integrate EFT into their daily routines for lasting results.

Case Study 1: Overcoming Stress and Anxiety

One of the most common uses of EFT is for managing stress and anxiety. Take the case of Sarah, a professional in her mid-30s who had been struggling with performance anxiety at work. Despite being competent in her job, Sarah would often freeze during presentations or feel an overwhelming sense of dread before meetings. This anxiety stemmed from a deep-rooted fear of making mistakes, which had built up over years of academic and professional pressure.

After working with an EFT practitioner, Sarah began using tapping techniques to address her anxiety. She focused on the emotions tied to her fear of failure, saying statements like, "Even though I feel terrified about making a mistake, I choose to feel calm and confident." Over time, Sarah's anxiety diminished, and she was able to enter meetings and presentations with a sense of ease. Her ability to process emotions in the moment, rather than letting them overwhelm her, was key to her success.

Practical Advice for Stress and Anxiety Relief

To reduce stress and anxiety through EFT, start by identifying the specific emotions that are triggering your anxiety. Tap on these emotions while repeating statements that acknowledge the fear, but also affirm a sense of calm and control. For example: "Even though I feel anxious about this presentation, I choose to remain calm and confident." Repeat the tapping routine as necessary until you feel a shift in your emotional state.

Case Study 2: Healing from Trauma

EFT has also shown great promise in helping individuals process and heal from trauma. John, a veteran of the military, had been dealing with post-traumatic stress disorder (PTSD) for years following his service. He had vivid flashbacks, nightmares, and severe anxiety whenever he encountered certain triggers. His relationship with his family had been affected, as he struggled with anger outbursts and emotional numbness.

Working with an EFT practitioner, John began tapping on the memories of his traumatic experiences. He started with the most distressing memories, focusing on the emotions they stirred—fear, helplessness, and anger. Using phrases like, "Even though I feel terrified and helpless when I think about what happened, I choose to release this fear and find peace," John gradually noticed a reduction in the intensity of his symptoms. Over the course of several weeks, his nightmares became less frequent, and he began to feel more emotionally present in his relationships.

Practical Advice for Trauma Recovery

For individuals dealing with trauma, EFT can be a powerful tool to release emotional charge and reprocess memories. It's important to work with a trained EFT practitioner when dealing with severe trauma to ensure that the process is handled safely. However, for less intense memories or emotional triggers, you can begin tapping by focusing on the emotions you feel when thinking about the traumatic event. Use statements like, "Even though I feel hurt/angry/sad when I remember this, I choose to let go of this pain and feel safe."

Case Study 3: Improving Relationships

EFT is not only useful for individuals but can also be applied in relationships to resolve conflicts, increase empathy, and improve communication. Lisa and Mark, a married couple, were experiencing ongoing communication issues, especially around finances and household responsibilities. They found themselves arguing frequently, each feeling unheard and misunderstood.

After learning EFT, Lisa and Mark began to tap together when they felt emotionally triggered during a disagreement. They focused on their individual feelings and used EFT to calm their emotional responses before continuing the conversation. By tapping on phrases like, "Even though I feel frustrated and unheard, I choose to stay calm and listen to my partner's perspective," both Lisa and Mark began to feel more emotionally connected and open to each other's viewpoints.

As they continued using EFT during their conflicts, the couple noticed that their arguments became less heated, and they started to address issues more constructively. They began using tapping not only during conflicts but also as a way to maintain emotional balance and enhance their overall communication.

Practical Advice for Relationship Conflicts

To use EFT in relationships, tap together as a couple when tensions arise. Focus on the emotions that come up during the conflict, such as frustration, fear, or hurt. Use tapping statements like, "Even though I feel hurt by what was said, I choose to stay open and communicate my feelings calmly." Over time, this will help reduce emotional reactivity and create a space for healthier, more empathetic communication.

Case Study 4: Addressing Phobias and Fears

Phobias are another area where EFT has shown success. Emma, a young woman with a severe fear of flying, had avoided air travel for years. Her fear was so intense that even the thought of boarding a plane triggered a panic attack. After a few EFT sessions, Emma learned how to tap on her fear and anxiety surrounding flying. She focused on specific thoughts like, "Even though I'm terrified of flying and feel completely out of control, I choose to feel calm and safe on a plane."

With regular EFT practice, Emma's fear began to subside. She was able to take a short flight for the first time in years, feeling calm and centered. Although her fear didn't disappear overnight, the tapping helped her to reduce the anxiety enough to take manageable steps toward overcoming the phobia.

Practical Advice for Phobias

If you are dealing with a phobia, identify the specific situations or thoughts that trigger your fear. Tap on those specific feelings, using statements like, "Even though I feel scared when I think about [the feared situation], I choose to release this fear and feel calm." With consistent tapping, the emotional intensity of the phobia should decrease over time, allowing you to feel more in control.

Case Study 5: Enhancing Personal Growth

EFT can also be used for personal development, helping individuals overcome limiting beliefs or achieve goals that seem out of reach. Tom, a successful entrepreneur, had always struggled with imposter syndrome. Despite his success, he felt unworthy of his accomplishments and feared that others would eventually discover that he wasn't "good enough." This fear held him back from taking bigger risks and expanding his business.

Through EFT, Tom learned to tap on these feelings of inadequacy. He focused on statements like, "Even though I feel like I don't deserve my success, I choose to release this belief and embrace my accomplishments." Over time, he began to feel more confident in his abilities and started taking the risks necessary to grow his business. EFT helped Tom replace limiting beliefs with empowering ones, allowing him to step into his full potential.

Practical Advice for Personal Growth

To use EFT for personal development, focus on the limiting beliefs or fears that are holding you back. Tap on those beliefs while repeating affirmations like, "Even though I believe I'm not capable of [achieving a goal], I choose to feel confident and capable." Regular tapping can help you break free from these self-imposed limitations and achieve your full potential.

Case studies demonstrate the wide range of issues that EFT can help address, from stress and anxiety to trauma, phobias, and relationship challenges. The beauty of EFT lies in its simplicity and versatility—it can be used alone or with a practitioner, and it can be tailored to fit individual needs. By tapping on emotional triggers, releasing negative feelings, and shifting limiting beliefs, EFT provides a powerful tool for emotional healing and personal growth. With consistent practice, it's possible to reduce emotional reactivity, improve relationships, and achieve greater emotional balance.

Self-love and acceptance are foundational to emotional well-being, yet many people struggle with feelings of inadequacy, low self-worth, or self-criticism. These feelings can stem from past experiences, societal pressures, or ingrained negative beliefs about oneself. Emotional Freedom Technique (EFT) offers a powerful tool to help individuals break free from these patterns by addressing emotional blockages and shifting negative beliefs. Through the practice of tapping, EFT facilitates a deeper connection to self-compassion and acceptance.

Understanding the Link Between Self-Love and Emotional Health

At the core of self-love and self-acceptance lies the ability to embrace one's flaws and strengths without judgment. When individuals struggle with self-worth, they often experience a cycle of self-criticism, anxiety, and even depression. These emotions are tied to a person's energy system and can block the natural flow of positive energy and self-compassion. EFT works by tapping on acupressure points to release the emotional charge associated with negative beliefs, allowing individuals to restore emotional balance and foster a healthier, more loving relationship with themselves.

How EFT Can Help Build Self-Love

EFT helps individuals clear emotional blockages that prevent self-love and acceptance. When practicing EFT for self-love, the focus is on identifying and addressing the negative self-beliefs or past experiences that contribute to low self-esteem. Common issues might include feelings of being "not good enough," fear of rejection, or guilt over past mistakes. These negative beliefs are often deep-seated and can take years to overcome through traditional self-help methods, but EFT can offer a quicker way to shift the emotional energy and thought patterns.

During an EFT session, individuals tap on a series of acupressure points while repeating statements that acknowledge their feelings and offer self-compassion. For example, someone who struggles with self-criticism might tap while saying, "Even though I don't feel good enough, I choose to love and accept myself as I am." This combination of physical tapping and emotional focus helps to release the negative charge associated with those beliefs, creating space for healthier, more supportive thoughts.

1. **Fear of Rejection or Abandonment**: Many individuals fear rejection, whether from a romantic partner, friends, or even their family. This fear can create a barrier to self-love, as it often leads to people seeking validation from others to feel worthy. EFT can address these feelings by tapping on the belief, "Even though I fear being rejected or abandoned, I choose to feel safe and secure in who I am."
2. **Guilt and Shame**: Guilt and shame are powerful emotions that can prevent individuals from accepting themselves. These feelings often arise from past actions or perceived mistakes, leading to self-criticism. By tapping on statements like, "Even though I feel guilty about [this past event], I choose to forgive myself and embrace my imperfections," individuals can begin to release the hold that guilt and shame have on their sense of self.
3. **Comparing Yourself to Others**: Social comparisons, especially in the age of social media, can foster feelings of inadequacy. EFT can help individuals address the belief that they aren't as good as others by tapping on statements such as, "Even though I compare myself to others and feel less than, I choose to accept myself for who I am."
4. **Perfectionism**: Perfectionism can make it difficult for individuals to feel good enough, as they are constantly striving for an unattainable standard. EFT can help by focusing on releasing the emotional charge around perfectionism. A tapping statement might include, "Even though I feel like I'm not enough unless I'm perfect, I choose to love myself unconditionally, flaws and all."

When using EFT to promote self-love, the goal is to replace negative self-talk with affirmations of acceptance and self-compassion. Some effective tapping statements might include:

- "Even though I feel unworthy of love, I choose to believe in my own value."
- "Even though I feel like I'm not enough, I accept myself just as I am."
- "Even though I've made mistakes, I choose to forgive myself and move forward."
- "Even though I fear rejection, I choose to trust that I am deserving of love and respect."
- "Even though I have a hard time loving myself, I choose to treat myself with kindness."

The key is to focus on the emotions behind the negative beliefs and tap while repeating statements that honor those feelings but gently encourage a shift toward more positive, loving thoughts.

The Role of EFT in Overcoming Negative Self-Talk

Negative self-talk is a significant barrier to self-love. When individuals are constantly criticizing themselves or engaging in internal dialogues that reinforce feelings of inadequacy, it can be challenging to break free from these patterns. EFT helps to break the cycle of negative self-talk by allowing individuals to address the underlying emotions and beliefs driving these thoughts.

For example, someone who often tells themselves, "I'm not good enough" may feel a deep sense of unworthiness. Tapping on this belief while saying, "Even though I feel like I'm not good enough, I choose to love and accept myself fully," can help release the emotional charge around this thought. As the individual taps, they begin to change the way they respond to their inner critic, replacing self-judgment with self-compassion.

EFT and Healing Childhood Wounds

Many issues related to self-love stem from childhood experiences, such as criticism from parents, bullying at school, or abandonment. These wounds can create lasting emotional scars that hinder self-acceptance. EFT is particularly effective in addressing these early wounds, as it helps individuals revisit these painful memories and release the emotional charge associated with them.

For example, an individual who was constantly criticized as a child may carry the belief that they are not good enough. Through EFT, the person can tap while focusing on the feelings connected to those childhood memories, saying, "Even though I was criticized as a child, I choose to release this pain and embrace my worth." This process helps to heal old wounds, allowing for greater self-compassion and self-love in the present.

EFT for Daily Practice of Self-Love

Incorporating EFT into a daily self-care routine can reinforce self-love and acceptance. A simple practice could involve tapping for a few minutes each morning or evening while focusing on positive affirmations. Tapping while saying statements like, "Even though I may have doubts, I choose to love and accept myself" or "Even though I have areas I want to improve, I am proud of how far I've come" can help set a positive tone for the day or promote relaxation before sleep.

For individuals who feel they don't have time for long sessions, EFT can be practiced in short bursts throughout the day. Tapping when feeling stressed, self-critical, or overwhelmed can immediately release negative emotions and reset the emotional state.

Over time, this regular practice can build a deeper connection to self-love and a more compassionate inner dialogue.

By consistently using EFT to address self-criticism, limiting beliefs, and emotional pain, individuals can experience lasting benefits in terms of self-love and acceptance. Over time, EFT helps to rewire the emotional patterns that no longer serve a person's well-being, creating a more positive and empowering relationship with oneself.

As emotional blockages are cleared, the individual can replace feelings of inadequacy with self-compassion and confidence. This, in turn, leads to improved mental health, greater resilience, and a more fulfilling life overall.

EFT offers a transformative approach to building self-love and acceptance. By tapping on emotional blocks, limiting beliefs, and negative self-talk, individuals can release the emotional charge associated with feelings of unworthiness and open themselves to the possibility of unconditional self-compassion. Whether addressing childhood wounds, perfectionism, or social comparisons, EFT helps individuals reconnect with their inherent value and worth. With regular practice, EFT can pave the way for a deeper sense of self-love, emotional balance, and inner peace.

Self-love is a crucial aspect of emotional well-being, yet many people struggle to cultivate a loving relationship with themselves due to deep-seated negative beliefs, past traumas, or societal pressures. Emotional Freedom Technique (EFT) can be a powerful tool to help individuals overcome these obstacles, release negative emotions, and foster greater self-compassion. By tapping on acupressure points while focusing on emotional challenges and using affirmations, EFT can break down the mental barriers preventing self-love and encourage positive, supportive feelings toward oneself.

EFT Tapping Techniques for Self-Love

To practice EFT for self-love, you begin by tapping on specific acupressure points while focusing on the negative emotions or beliefs that prevent you from fully accepting and loving yourself. The combination of physical tapping and verbal affirmation can create a sense of emotional release, gradually shifting your mindset from self-criticism to self-compassion. Here's a guide to some effective EFT techniques:

1. Identifying the Negative Self-Beliefs

The first step in any EFT session for self-love is identifying the beliefs or emotions that need to be addressed. This might include feelings like "I'm not good enough," "I'm unworthy of love," or "I'll never be able to love myself." These beliefs often come from past experiences, trauma, or societal conditioning. When tapping, it's important to start with these negative beliefs and emotions to address the root causes of low self-esteem.

Example: If you have a belief like "I'm not worthy of love," you would begin tapping while acknowledging this thought, using phrases such as:

- "Even though I feel like I'm not worthy of love, I choose to love and accept myself."
- "Even though I have this belief that I'm unworthy, I am open to releasing it now."

2. The Basic EFT Tapping Points

EFT uses a sequence of acupressure points that are gently tapped while focusing on the negative emotion or belief. The common tapping points are:

- **Karate Chop Point**: On the side of your hand, used for the setup statement.
- **Top of the Head**: Directly on the crown of your head.
- **Eyebrow**: Just above the nose, at the beginning of the eyebrow.
- **Side of the Eye**: On the bone at the outside corner of your eye.
- **Under the Eye**: On the bone just below the eye.
- **Under the Nose**: In the indentation between the nose and upper lip.
- **Chin**: In the indentation between your lower lip and chin.
- **Collarbone**: Just below the collarbone, on either side of the chest.
- **Under the Arm**: About 4 inches below the armpit.

For self-love, start by tapping on the **Karate Chop point** while saying the setup phrase. Then, move through the other points, tapping gently while repeating reminder phrases.

3. Tapping Phrases for Self-Love

The key to EFT is using the right statements that align with the issue you're addressing. When working on self-love, your goal is to acknowledge the negative belief but then shift it toward acceptance, love, and compassion. Here are some useful tapping statements:

- "Even though I don't love myself the way I want to, I deeply and completely love and accept myself."
- "Even though I feel unworthy of love, I choose to love and accept myself fully."
- "Even though I feel like I'm not good enough, I choose to embrace my worth and love myself unconditionally."
- "Even though I've made mistakes, I choose to forgive myself and love who I am today."
- "Even though I have a hard time accepting myself, I choose to release this resistance and open my heart to self-love."

The idea is to start with the problem or feeling you're working through but end with a positive affirmation that reaffirms self-acceptance and love.

4. Focusing on Specific Issues

If you know the specific areas of your life or self-perception where you struggle with self-love, you can tailor your tapping to these issues. For example:

- **Body Image Issues**: "Even though I don't like my body, I choose to appreciate it for all it does for me."
- **Fear of Rejection**: "Even though I fear being rejected, I choose to love myself regardless of others' opinions."
- **Perfectionism**: "Even though I feel I'm not good enough unless I'm perfect, I choose to love myself with all my flaws."

By targeting the exact issue, EFT helps release the emotional charge tied to it, allowing for deeper healing.

5. Using Affirmations to Reinforce Self-Love

Once you've worked through the negative beliefs with EFT, it's helpful to finish your session with positive affirmations that reinforce your self-worth and love. These affirmations can be repeated during the tapping process or as a standalone practice afterward.

Affirmations for Self-Love:

- "I am deserving of love and happiness."
- "I love and accept myself exactly as I am."
- "I am enough, just as I am."
- "I forgive myself for past mistakes and embrace my growth."
- "I choose to honor and cherish myself every day."

6. Using EFT to Let Go of Past Trauma

Many individuals struggle with self-love because of past trauma, whether it's emotional, physical, or verbal abuse, or other negative experiences. EFT can be used to target these past memories and release the emotional charge associated with them. You would focus on the specific memory, and use tapping statements like:

- "Even though I went through [specific event], I choose to forgive myself and release the pain."
- "Even though I was hurt in the past, I choose to love and accept myself now."

Over time, as you release the emotional pain attached to these memories, you'll begin to see yourself in a more loving and compassionate light.

For lasting results, consider incorporating EFT into your daily routine. Whether it's a brief tapping session each morning or taking a few minutes before bed to focus on self-love, regular practice will help reinforce your positive beliefs and build a stronger connection to self-compassion. A daily session can also help reset your emotional state when negative thoughts about yourself arise, allowing you to respond with self-love rather than self-criticism.

Daily Tapping Routine Example:

1. Start by identifying any negative thoughts or feelings you're holding about yourself that day.
2. Tap through the points while repeating statements like: "Even though I feel [emotion], I choose to love myself fully."
3. After the negative emotions subside, finish with positive affirmations like: "I am worthy of love and respect," "I am enough just as I am."

To deepen the self-love experience, you can pair EFT with visualization techniques. After tapping on the negative feelings and beliefs, take a moment to visualize yourself surrounded by love and compassion. Picture yourself accepting and embracing all aspects of who you are, and see yourself radiating self-confidence and joy. This visual reinforcement, combined with EFT, can help anchor the feelings of self-love on a deeper level.

EFT is a simple yet powerful technique that can help individuals overcome self-doubt, negative beliefs, and past trauma, and cultivate a loving, accepting relationship with themselves. By tapping on the acupressure points while focusing on self-love affirmations, individuals can release emotional blockages and transform their mindset. Over time, regular use of EFT can lead to a deeper connection with self-compassion, improved self-esteem, and a lasting sense of inner peace and acceptance. Whether you're working through deep-rooted emotional wounds or simply seeking to enhance your self-love, EFT offers a practical, accessible path to emotional healing.

Incorporating Emotional Freedom Technique (EFT) into your daily routine can be a transformative way to manage stress, improve emotional well-being, and foster a more positive mindset. EFT is a simple yet powerful tool that involves tapping on specific acupressure points on the body while focusing on the emotions or thoughts you want to release. With consistent practice, it can become a natural part of your life, helping you to navigate challenges with greater emotional resilience and self-awareness. Here are some practical ways to integrate EFT into your daily routine.

1. Morning Ritual for Setting Intentions

Starting your day with a short EFT session can help set a positive tone and prepare you mentally for the day ahead. As soon as you wake up, take a few moments to identify how you're feeling. Are you feeling stressed, anxious, or energized? Use EFT to address any negative emotions or self-doubt that may arise in the morning.

Example:
If you're feeling anxious about the day ahead, begin by tapping on the **Karate Chop point** (the side of your hand) and say something like, "Even though I feel anxious about the day ahead, I choose to feel calm and focused." Then, tap through the standard points (eyebrow, side of the eye, under the eye, etc.) while repeating this affirmation. This practice helps to clear any anxiety, leaving you feeling centered and ready to tackle the day with confidence.

2. Midday Break to Reconnect

Life can get overwhelming, and stress tends to build up throughout the day, especially in busy work or school environments. Taking a break to tap during the afternoon can help reset your emotional state, release accumulated stress, and refresh your mind.

Example:
When you start to feel stressed, frustrated, or fatigued, take a 5-minute break to do a quick EFT session. Focus on the stress you're experiencing and use tapping to release it. For instance, "Even though I feel overwhelmed by my to-do list, I choose to release this stress and feel clear and focused." You can also tap while focusing on something you want to feel, such as productivity or calmness. This can help you regain emotional balance and keep you focused for the remainder of the day.

3. Tapping During Emotional Moments

One of the easiest ways to incorporate EFT into your daily routine is to use it as a tool during emotional moments. Whether you're feeling frustrated, sad, angry, or even joyful, tapping can help you process and release emotions, allowing you to stay emotionally grounded throughout the day.

Example:

If a difficult situation arises—whether it's an argument with a colleague, a frustrating task, or a moment of self-doubt—stop for a moment to tap. Focus on the emotions you're feeling and tap while saying, "Even though I feel upset (or whatever emotion you're feeling), I choose to release this and feel more at ease." This allows you to process the emotions in real-time, reducing their intensity and preventing them from lingering or escalating.

4. Evening Practice for Reflection and Relaxation

Before bed is a great time to incorporate EFT into your routine, as it can help you wind down and release any negative emotions or thoughts from the day. This can also help prevent stress or anxiety from affecting your sleep. Taking time to tap and reflect on the day allows you to process any lingering emotions, clearing your mind before resting.

Example:

As part of your bedtime routine, sit comfortably and focus on the feelings you've experienced throughout the day. You can tap on any lingering stress or emotions that need to be released. For instance, "Even though I feel unsettled by today's events, I choose to release this tension and relax completely." After tapping, you might feel more relaxed, centered, and ready for a restful night's sleep.

5. Tapping to Build Positive Habits

Incorporating EFT into your daily routine can also support the development of positive habits, such as boosting self-confidence, motivation, or positive thinking. Whether you want to foster gratitude, self-love, or optimism, EFT can help shift your mindset in a positive direction.

Example:

If you're trying to build a new habit, like exercising more or eating healthier, you can tap on your motivation to help reinforce the behavior. Say something like, "Even though I've struggled with staying consistent, I choose to embrace this new habit and feel energized and motivated." Tapping in this way helps to remove the emotional resistance to change and reinforce your commitment to your goals.

6. Tapping for Physical Symptoms

EFT isn't just effective for emotional issues; it can also be a helpful tool for managing physical symptoms that arise throughout the day, like tension headaches, muscle pain, or digestive discomfort. If you notice physical discomfort, tapping can help release the stress or emotions associated with the pain.

Example:

If you're experiencing a headache, focus on the sensation while tapping. Start by saying, "Even though I have this headache, I choose to release the tension and feel comfortable." Tap through the points while focusing on the physical sensation, and with repeated practice, you may find the pain lessens or disappears.

7. Tapping in the Moment of Crisis

Sometimes, life's unexpected challenges or emotional moments can catch you off guard. In such moments, EFT can be used quickly and discreetly to regain composure and regain emotional balance. This is particularly helpful in situations like arguments, emotional overwhelm, or stressful encounters.

Example:

If you're feeling overwhelmed in a social setting or during a challenging conversation, take a moment to tap on the side of your hand (Karate Chop point) and say, "Even though I feel overwhelmed right now, I choose to stay calm and centered." Tap through the points while focusing on staying grounded. This will help you manage your emotional reaction and regain clarity in the moment.

8. Using EFT to Affirmations for Daily Growth

Another great way to incorporate EFT into your day is by combining it with affirmations for personal growth. While tapping through the points, you can affirm qualities such as confidence, self-love, and success.

Example:

Say affirmations like, "Even though I sometimes doubt myself, I choose to believe in my abilities," or "Even though I feel uncertain, I trust that I am on the right path." Tapping while repeating these affirmations can reinforce positive beliefs and help you foster a mindset of growth and resilience.

Incorporating EFT into your daily routine offers numerous benefits for emotional regulation, stress relief, and personal development. Whether used in the morning to set a positive tone for the day, during stressful moments to release emotional charges, or before bed to unwind and reflect, EFT provides a simple yet effective method to improve emotional well-being and stay centered. By making EFT a consistent part of your routine, you can enhance your resilience, improve your emotional health, and foster a greater sense of peace throughout your day.

Personal development often involves overcoming internal barriers and limiting beliefs that hold individuals back from reaching their full potential. Emotional Freedom Technique (EFT) has emerged as a transformative tool for people seeking personal growth, offering a way to release emotional blocks and adopt a more positive mindset. Many individuals have shared inspiring stories of how EFT has played a crucial role in their journeys of self-improvement, from overcoming fear and self-doubt to achieving career success and improving relationships.

Overcoming Fear of Public Speaking

One of the most common challenges people face in personal development is overcoming the fear of public speaking. This fear, known as glossophobia, affects millions of people and can limit their career and personal growth. For a woman named Sarah, this fear was a significant barrier to her career advancement. Despite her talent and expertise, she found herself avoiding presentations and meetings, worried about making mistakes or being judged by her peers.

Sarah decided to try EFT after hearing about its potential to address deep-seated fears and anxieties. She began by tapping on the **Karate Chop** point while acknowledging her fear, saying, "Even though I'm terrified of speaking in public, I choose to feel calm and confident." She continued tapping on the standard points while repeating this affirmation.

After several EFT sessions, Sarah noticed a dramatic shift in her mindset. The intense fear that once paralyzed her during presentations gradually diminished. She no longer feared judgment or mistakes, allowing her to focus on the content of her presentations rather than her own anxiety. With increased confidence, Sarah went on to secure a promotion and even volunteered to give a keynote speech at an industry conference.

Building Self-Esteem and Confidence

Another common area of personal development where EFT has proven effective is in improving self-esteem. John, a man in his late 30s, had struggled with low self-esteem for most of his life. Growing up in a critical household, he internalized negative messages about his worth, leading him to feel inadequate in both his personal and professional life. As an adult, he found it difficult to assert himself in relationships and often second-guessed his decisions.

John turned to EFT in an attempt to break free from the cycle of self-criticism. He started with tapping on the **Karate Chop** point while acknowledging his feelings of low self-worth: "Even though I don't feel good enough, I choose to accept and love myself." He then tapped through the standard points while repeating affirmations such as, "I am worthy of success and happiness," and "I trust my decisions."

Over the course of a few weeks, John noticed a significant shift in his self-perception. He became more confident in his abilities and felt less anxious about making mistakes. His improved self-esteem positively impacted his career, allowing him to take on new challenges and build stronger, more confident relationships. EFT helped him unlock the belief that he was deserving of love and success, which had previously been a barrier to his personal growth.

Letting Go of Past Trauma

Personal development often requires individuals to confront and heal from past emotional wounds. For Maria, an entrepreneur in her early 40s, unresolved trauma from her childhood had kept her stuck in unhealthy relationship patterns and held her back from fully embracing her potential. Maria had suffered emotional abuse from a close family member, which had left deep scars on her sense of self-worth. As an adult, she found it difficult to trust others and often sabotaged relationships before they could grow too serious.

Maria began using EFT to address the deep-seated pain from her past. She started by focusing on the traumatic memories that triggered feelings of unworthiness and fear of abandonment. She tapped on the **Karate Chop** point while saying, "Even though I was hurt by someone I loved, I choose to release this pain and open my heart to healing." She continued tapping through the points while visualizing herself letting go of the emotional baggage tied to her past.

After several sessions, Maria began to feel lighter and more empowered. The negative emotions tied to her past trauma no longer had the same hold over her, and she was able to build healthier relationships. EFT helped her release the emotional charge associated with the trauma, allowing her to embrace a future of love, trust, and personal fulfillment. Maria's journey of healing is a powerful testament to how EFT can support the process of overcoming emotional wounds and reclaiming one's personal power.

Achieving Career Success

For many individuals, career growth is a key component of personal development. Michael, a graphic designer in his early 30s, felt like he was stuck in a professional rut. Despite having the skills and experience to advance, he struggled with self-doubt and the fear that he wasn't good enough to compete with more seasoned professionals. He found himself procrastinating on important projects and turning down opportunities that could have propelled his career forward.

Michael decided to use EFT to address the mental blocks that were hindering his career. He began by tapping on the **Karate Chop** point while acknowledging his fears of inadequacy: "Even though I feel like I'm not skilled enough, I choose to believe in my abilities." After a few weeks of tapping daily, Michael felt a noticeable shift in his confidence. He no longer procrastinated or avoided opportunities, and he started pursuing bigger projects with excitement rather than anxiety.

With increased confidence, Michael approached his career with renewed enthusiasm and clarity. He took on higher-profile clients, developed his portfolio, and even started teaching design workshops. EFT helped him release the limiting beliefs that had held him back, opening up new opportunities and allowing him to thrive professionally.

Improving Relationships Through EFT

Personal development is often deeply intertwined with the quality of our relationships. For Lisa, a woman in her mid-40s, EFT played a pivotal role in improving both her romantic and familial relationships. Lisa had a history of attracting emotionally unavailable partners, and she struggled to communicate her needs in her family relationships. She realized that unresolved childhood issues and past heartbreaks were affecting her ability to form healthy, balanced relationships.

Lisa began using EFT to address these issues, focusing on the fear of rejection and the belief that she wasn't worthy of a loving, fulfilling relationship. She tapped on the **Karate Chop** point while saying, "Even though I fear being rejected, I choose to let go of this fear and embrace the love I deserve." She also tapped on issues from her past, such as unresolved conflicts with her parents, using the phrase, "Even though I have unresolved issues with my parents, I choose to release these wounds and move forward with love."

As Lisa continued her EFT practice, she noticed profound changes in how she approached relationships. She became more open, communicative, and willing to set healthy boundaries. Her relationship with her partner improved significantly, and she began to form deeper, more meaningful connections with her family members.

These personal development stories illustrate how EFT can be a powerful tool for overcoming emotional blocks, shifting limiting beliefs, and fostering positive change in various areas of life. Whether it's addressing fears, improving self-esteem, letting go of past trauma, advancing in a career, or enhancing relationships, EFT offers a practical, accessible method for self-growth. The stories of Sarah, John, Maria, Michael, and Lisa demonstrate the transformative potential of EFT when used consistently to address emotional challenges and support personal development. With the right mindset and dedication, EFT can help anyone unlock their full potential and create lasting, positive change.

EFT for Physical Pain and Healing

Physical pain, whether acute or chronic, can have a significant impact on a person's quality of life. While many people rely on traditional medical treatments for relief, a growing number are turning to alternative methods like Emotional Freedom Technique (EFT) to complement their healing process. EFT, often referred to as "tapping," is a form of psychological acupressure that targets specific energy points on the body while focusing on emotions or pain. Research and anecdotal evidence suggest that EFT can help reduce both physical pain and the emotional components that often accompany it.

The Mind-Body Connection

One of the central concepts in EFT is the understanding of the mind-body connection. Research has long established that emotional stress, unresolved trauma, and negative thought patterns can manifest physically in the body. This can lead to chronic pain, tension, and discomfort. Conditions like fibromyalgia, migraines, back pain, and joint issues often have emotional triggers or psychological components that contribute to the intensity of the pain.

EFT works on the premise that when the body's energy system is disrupted by negative emotions, physical pain can arise. By tapping on specific acupressure points on the body, EFT aims to restore balance to the energy system, release emotional blockages, and reduce the intensity of physical pain. This dual focus on emotional and physical well-being makes EFT a holistic approach to pain management.

How EFT Can Help with Physical Pain

1. Reducing Muscle Tension

Chronic pain often leads to muscle tension, which can create a cycle of discomfort. For example, someone with a history of neck and shoulder pain may find that stress and anxiety exacerbate the tension, making the pain worse. EFT can help break this cycle by addressing both the emotional triggers that cause stress and the physical symptoms that result from it. Tapping on the energy points while focusing on the discomfort can send a signal to the brain to relax, allowing the body to release stored tension.

Example:
If you're experiencing neck pain, start by tapping on the **Karate Chop point** (the side of

the hand) and say, "Even though I feel tightness and pain in my neck, I choose to relax and release this tension." Tap through the rest of the energy points while focusing on the pain and repeating your affirmation. Many users report a noticeable reduction in muscle tightness after a few rounds of tapping.

2. Alleviating Chronic Pain

For people suffering from chronic pain, EFT offers a way to manage and reduce pain intensity. Chronic pain conditions such as arthritis, fibromyalgia, or lower back pain can often be improved through regular EFT practice. In these cases, it is crucial to focus both on the physical pain and the emotional aspect of the pain.

Example:
A person with lower back pain might tap on the **Top of the Head** while saying, "Even though I have this pain in my lower back, I choose to feel relief and comfort." The tapping process helps the person confront not just the pain but also any negative emotions associated with it, such as fear, frustration, or helplessness. By repeatedly tapping and focusing on the pain, many find their chronic pain lessens in intensity over time.

3. Emotional Triggers for Pain

In some cases, physical pain is directly linked to unresolved emotions or past trauma. Emotional events, whether they occur in childhood or adulthood, can become "trapped" in the body and manifest as physical discomfort. EFT can help release these emotional blocks and, in turn, reduce the physical pain caused by them.

Example:
A person with long-term knee pain may tap on the **Eyebrow** point while saying, "Even though I've been carrying emotional pain in my knees, I choose to release the past and allow healing." As the tapping continues, the person may start to recognize that the pain is not just physical but is also connected to feelings of being stuck or unable to move forward in life. By addressing these emotions during the tapping process, the pain may begin to dissipate, and healing can take place.

Combining EFT with Traditional Pain Management

Many individuals find that combining EFT with traditional pain management techniques enhances their overall well-being. EFT can be used alongside physical therapies, medication, or other holistic methods to amplify the effects of treatment. For example, someone undergoing physical therapy for knee pain might practice EFT before or after their sessions to help reduce stress, calm the nervous system, and release any emotional resistance to healing.

Example:
After receiving physical therapy for knee rehabilitation, a person could tap on the **Side of the Eye** and say, "Even though this rehab is challenging, I choose to feel strong and open to healing." This mindset shift can allow the body to respond more positively to physical treatments, reducing the psychological stress associated with recovery.

Case Studies and Success Stories

Numerous individuals have reported success with EFT for managing physical pain, from acute injuries to chronic conditions. A study on the effectiveness of EFT for chronic pain found that participants who combined EFT with other treatments experienced significant reductions in pain intensity and emotional distress. One participant, suffering from chronic back pain, used EFT in combination with physical therapy and reported a 50% reduction in pain after just a few sessions.

Similarly, individuals with conditions like fibromyalgia have shared success stories of how EFT helped alleviate both pain and the emotional struggles that often accompany the condition. These stories often highlight the importance of addressing the emotional component of physical pain, showing how EFT not only reduces pain but also improves quality of life by helping individuals feel more empowered in their healing journey.

The Science Behind EFT for Pain

While more research is needed to fully understand the mechanisms behind EFT, several studies have provided evidence of its effectiveness for pain relief. One study published in the "Journal of Nervous and Mental Disease" showed that EFT reduced pain intensity in patients with fibromyalgia, with participants reporting an average reduction of 41% in pain after just one session. Other research has found that EFT helps regulate the body's stress response, reducing cortisol levels and promoting relaxation, which can contribute to reduced pain perception.

EFT is also believed to work by addressing the body's energy system, similar to traditional acupuncture. The theory is that tapping on acupressure points stimulates the body's energy flow, helping to unblock energy that may be contributing to pain. This mechanism, combined with the psychological effects of tapping, offers a holistic approach to pain management.

Final Thoughts

EFT provides a versatile and effective tool for managing physical pain and promoting healing. By addressing both the emotional and physical aspects of pain, it can complement traditional treatments and help individuals achieve lasting relief. Whether it's used to alleviate muscle tension, reduce chronic pain, or heal emotional wounds tied to physical discomfort, EFT offers a non-invasive and accessible option for those seeking alternative or supplementary pain management strategies. As more people discover the power of EFT, it continues to gain recognition as a powerful tool for promoting overall well-being and healing.

Understanding the mind-body connection

The mind and body are intricately connected, with each influencing the other in ways that are still being explored by modern science. While the physical body can affect mental health, such as when pain or illness leads to depression or anxiety, the reverse is also true: mental states like stress, anger, and fear can manifest as physical ailments. Emotional Freedom Technique (EFT) leverages this mind-body connection by addressing emotional issues that may be causing physical discomfort or illness. Through the tapping of acupressure points on the body, EFT seeks to restore balance to the energy system, alleviate emotional distress, and promote physical healing.

The Concept of Energy in the Body

In traditional Eastern medicine, it is believed that the body's vital energy flows through a network of pathways, often referred to as meridians. When this energy flow is disrupted or blocked—due to stress, trauma, or negative emotions—physical or emotional symptoms can arise. These disruptions in the energy system can contribute to a range of issues, from chronic pain to anxiety, depression, or even serious illnesses.

EFT works on the premise that by stimulating specific acupressure points while focusing on emotional or physical concerns, a person can restore the flow of energy through the meridians. The tapping process sends signals to the brain, helping to calm the nervous system and release any negative emotions or blocks that may be contributing to physical pain or emotional distress. The theory is that when the mind and body are in alignment, and when energy flows freely, both emotional and physical health improve.

How Emotions Influence Physical Health

Emotions have a profound impact on our physical health. The body's response to emotional stress can trigger physical reactions, such as muscle tension, headaches, or digestive issues. This is why emotional states like anxiety or anger are often linked to conditions such as migraines, back pain, or irritable bowel syndrome (IBS). Chronic stress, in particular, can weaken the immune system, increase inflammation, and lead to various health complications.

When we experience strong emotions, the body responds by releasing chemicals such as adrenaline and cortisol, commonly known as the stress hormones. While these chemicals are helpful in short bursts—helping us to fight or flee from danger—they can be harmful if they remain elevated for extended periods. Chronic emotional stress can lead to long-term health problems, including cardiovascular disease, digestive issues, and sleep disorders.

EFT helps break this cycle by addressing the emotional triggers that activate the body's stress response. By tapping on key energy points, EFT provides a way to calm the body and shift its reaction to emotional stimuli. The process allows individuals to release emotional charges associated with past trauma, current stress, or anxiety, helping to reduce the physical effects of those emotions.

The Role of EFT in Restoring the Mind-Body Balance

One of the key principles behind EFT is the idea that unresolved emotions are often stored in the body. These emotions can create "energy blocks" that prevent the body from functioning optimally. By addressing these blocks through tapping, EFT aims to restore balance to the body's energy system and, in turn, improve both emotional and physical well-being.

For example, someone dealing with chronic pain, such as back pain or headaches, may find that the pain is not only physical but also linked to emotional stress. In such cases, EFT can be used to target both the physical pain and the emotional issues that are contributing to it. When the emotional charge associated with the pain is reduced through tapping, the body may also experience a reduction in the intensity of the physical pain. This highlights how addressing emotional blockages can lead to improvements in physical health.

Addressing Emotional Trauma and Its Impact on the Body

Traumatic experiences, whether physical, emotional, or psychological, can have a lasting impact on the body. PTSD (Post-Traumatic Stress Disorder) is a clear example of how emotional trauma can affect both the mind and the body. People suffering from PTSD often experience physical symptoms such as muscle tension, headaches, or digestive problems, which are linked to the emotional distress caused by the trauma.

EFT can be particularly effective for individuals who are dealing with past trauma. By tapping on acupressure points while focusing on the emotional pain or memories associated with the trauma, EFT helps to release the negative emotional charge. Over time, this can lead to a significant reduction in the physical symptoms that are often associated with unresolved trauma.

Stress and the Nervous System

The autonomic nervous system, which regulates involuntary bodily functions such as heart rate and digestion, plays a key role in how the body responds to stress. When stress levels rise, the sympathetic nervous system (the "fight or flight" system) is activated, preparing the body for action. However, if stress is chronic, the body remains in a heightened state of alert, which can lead to physical problems such as high blood pressure, muscle tension, and digestive issues.

EFT helps to activate the parasympathetic nervous system, the "rest and digest" system, which counteracts the effects of stress. By tapping on specific acupressure points, EFT promotes a state of calm and relaxation, helping the body shift out of its stress response and return to a balanced, healing state. This can have immediate and long-lasting effects on both emotional and physical health.

Scientific Backing for EFT's Impact on the Mind-Body Connection

While EFT is still considered an alternative therapy, several scientific studies have demonstrated its effectiveness in reducing both emotional and physical symptoms. Research has shown that EFT can lower cortisol levels (a stress hormone), improve mood, reduce anxiety, and even decrease the intensity of pain. For example, a study published in the *Journal of Nervous and Mental Disease* found that individuals who received EFT treatment experienced a significant reduction in their pain levels, as well as a decrease in negative emotional states, such as anxiety and depression.

Other studies have explored EFT's impact on physical health conditions. One study on chronic pain found that EFT participants experienced a substantial reduction in pain intensity after just a few sessions. The research concluded that EFT could be an effective tool for managing pain by addressing both the emotional and physical aspects of the condition.

Understanding the mind-body connection is crucial for holistic health and well-being. Emotions are not merely psychological experiences; they have profound physical effects that can either promote healing or contribute to illness. EFT works by addressing the emotional underpinnings of physical pain and discomfort, offering a powerful tool for restoring balance to the mind and body. Through tapping on acupressure points, EFT helps release emotional blockages, calm the nervous system, and improve overall health. Whether used for managing stress, alleviating pain, or healing from trauma, EFT highlights the importance of integrating emotional well-being with physical health.

Pain is a complex experience that can be physical, emotional, or both. Traditional methods of pain relief often focus on the physical aspect—such as medication, surgery, or physical therapy—but increasingly, people are discovering the benefits of addressing the emotional and psychological factors that can contribute to or exacerbate pain. Emotional Freedom Technique (EFT), a form of energy psychology, offers an alternative approach to pain relief by combining tapping on acupressure points with psychological focus to reduce both emotional distress and physical discomfort.

The Science Behind EFT and Pain Relief

The body's energy system, which is similar to the concepts behind acupuncture, plays a key role in EFT. When we experience emotional distress, it is believed that the energy flow in the body becomes disrupted, leading to physical symptoms, including pain. EFT works by tapping on specific acupressure points while focusing on the pain or emotional issue. This tapping stimulates the body's energy system, helping to restore balance and reduce the intensity of both the emotional and physical experiences related to pain.

Many studies have shown that EFT can help lower stress levels, reduce inflammation, and decrease the emotional components of pain, which can, in turn, reduce physical discomfort. The key to EFT's effectiveness is its ability to address not only the pain itself but the underlying emotional triggers that may intensify it.

Basic EFT Technique for Pain Relief

To begin using EFT for pain relief, you can follow a basic tapping sequence. This sequence involves tapping on specific acupressure points on the body while repeating affirmations or statements related to the pain or discomfort. The basic tapping points are as follows:

1. **Karate Chop Point** (Side of the Hand): This point is used to begin the session and is often tapped while stating the problem.
2. **Top of the Head**: This point is located on the crown of the head.
3. **Eyebrow Point**: Located at the beginning of the eyebrow, just above the nose.
4. **Side of the Eye**: On the bone at the side of the eye.
5. **Under the Eye**: On the bone directly beneath the eye.
6. **Under the Nose**: The point located just below the nose and above the upper lip.
7. **Chin Point**: The area between the bottom of the lower lip and the chin.
8. **Collarbone Point**: Just below the collarbone, about an inch down from the center of the chest.
9. **Under the Arm**: About four inches below the armpit.

Step-by-Step Process for Tapping

1. **Identify the Pain**: Focus on the area of discomfort and identify the pain's intensity on a scale from 0 to 10, where 0 is no pain and 10 is the worst pain imaginable. This helps track your progress during the session.

2. **Set an Intention**: While tapping on the Karate Chop point, say a statement like, "Even though I have this [pain description], I deeply and completely accept myself." This affirmation is designed to acknowledge the pain and any related emotional issues without judgment.
3. **Tap Through the Points**: As you tap through each of the points, focus on the pain and continue to repeat phrases such as, "This pain in my [location] is here," or "I feel discomfort in my [location] and I'm ready to release it."
4. **Reassess**: After a round of tapping, assess the pain intensity again on a scale of 0 to 10. Many individuals report a decrease in pain after just a few rounds of tapping, though some may require more sessions to achieve lasting relief.

EFT for Chronic Pain

Chronic pain is particularly suited to EFT because it often involves both emotional and physical components. In chronic pain conditions such as fibromyalgia, arthritis, or migraines, emotional factors like stress, frustration, and fear can heighten the perception of pain. EFT helps break the cycle by addressing both the physical symptoms and the emotional triggers.

For example, someone with chronic back pain might tap on the side of the eye while saying, "Even though I've had this back pain for years, I choose to release the emotional tension that is holding it in place." This dual focus on emotional release and physical discomfort can bring a reduction in pain intensity and an increase in overall comfort.

EFT for Acute Pain

For acute pain, such as a sprained ankle or a headache, EFT can also be effective. The tapping process helps to reduce the body's stress response and can help lower the intensity of the pain in real-time.

Example:
If you have a headache, you might start tapping on the Karate Chop point while saying, "Even though I have this intense headache, I choose to relax and let go of the pain." Continue tapping through the points while focusing on the headache. With each round, many people notice a reduction in the severity of their pain.

Addressing Emotional Triggers of Pain

Pain, especially chronic pain, is often not just a physical sensation but a complex interplay of physical, emotional, and psychological factors. Past trauma, stress, and negative thought patterns can worsen the perception of pain. By addressing these emotional triggers, EFT can provide relief from the underlying emotional causes of the pain, allowing the body to heal.

Example:
Someone who has pain related to an old injury might tap while saying, "Even though I feel anger and frustration about this old injury, I'm willing to release these emotions and allow my body to heal." The emotional release that comes from tapping can help free the body from the emotional charge associated with past trauma, leading to less intense pain.

EFT for Pain Management: Real-Life Success Stories

Numerous individuals have used EFT successfully to manage both chronic and acute pain. A study on the effects of EFT for fibromyalgia, a condition marked by widespread musculoskeletal pain, found that participants who used EFT experienced significant reductions in both pain and emotional distress. Some participants reported pain reductions of over 50%, which they attributed to both the emotional relief from past traumas and the physical relaxation achieved through tapping.

Another real-life example is a person who used EFT for migraine relief. After several rounds of tapping, their migraine, which had been an 8 out of 10 on the pain scale, dropped to a 3. They continued to use tapping regularly, and over time, their migraine frequency and intensity decreased significantly.

Combining EFT with Other Pain Relief Strategies

While EFT can be a highly effective standalone treatment, it is often used in conjunction with other pain relief strategies. People may use EFT alongside medication, physical therapy, or relaxation techniques to enhance their overall pain management approach. This combination allows for a holistic approach to healing, addressing not just the physical symptoms but also the mental and emotional aspects of pain.

Final Thoughts

EFT offers a unique and effective approach to pain relief by addressing the complex mind-body connection that underlies both emotional and physical pain. Whether used for chronic conditions like arthritis and fibromyalgia or acute pain from injury, EFT provides a non-invasive and empowering method for managing discomfort. Through the simple technique of tapping on acupressure points while focusing on pain and related emotions, many individuals experience significant relief, making EFT a powerful tool for pain management and overall wellness.

Personal stories and case studies provide a powerful illustration of how Emotional Freedom Technique (EFT) can be transformative in addressing emotional, psychological, and physical issues. By combining acupressure with psychological focus, EFT helps individuals process and release emotional blockages, alleviating symptoms of stress, anxiety, pain, trauma, and more. Many people have experienced profound changes after incorporating EFT into their healing journey.

Case Study 1: Overcoming Chronic Pain

Janet, a 45-year-old woman, had been living with chronic back pain for over a decade. Despite undergoing various treatments, including physical therapy, medication, and even surgery, the pain persisted. During an EFT session, Janet focused on the emotional aspect of her pain, particularly the frustration she felt from not being able to live an active lifestyle. She started tapping on the acupressure points, voicing phrases like, "Even though I have this pain in my back, I deeply and completely accept myself."

After several rounds of tapping, Janet reported a noticeable reduction in her pain. By exploring the emotional connection to her pain—particularly feelings of helplessness and anger—she was able to release some of the emotional charge. Over time, Janet used EFT regularly to manage her pain and even noticed improvements in her overall mobility and mood. Her experience highlights how chronic pain is often linked to emotional factors, and addressing those through EFT can lead to significant relief.

Case Study 2: Reducing Anxiety and Panic Attacks

Carlos, a 30-year-old man, struggled with severe anxiety and panic attacks. The attacks were so intense that he had difficulty leaving his home, fearing the next episode could occur at any time. Carlos tried conventional therapy and medication, but the results were temporary.

After learning about EFT, he decided to try it. In his first session, Carlos focused on the specific triggers of his panic attacks, such as feeling trapped or overwhelmed in public spaces. As he tapped through the acupressure points, he repeated affirmations like, "Even though I feel trapped and scared in crowded places, I am safe and in control."

After just a few sessions, Carlos experienced a dramatic reduction in the frequency and intensity of his panic attacks. By acknowledging and processing the underlying emotions—such as fear of judgment and loss of control—Carlos felt empowered to face situations that had previously induced anxiety. His success with EFT led him to use the technique regularly as a tool for managing anxiety, and over time, his panic attacks diminished almost entirely.

Case Study 3: Healing from Trauma and PTSD

Sophia, a 50-year-old woman, had suffered from post-traumatic stress disorder (PTSD) due to a car accident she experienced years ago. The trauma had caused recurring nightmares, flashbacks, and intense emotional distress. Despite undergoing traditional therapies such as talk therapy and cognitive-behavioral therapy (CBT), Sophia found little relief.

Sophia decided to try EFT after hearing about its success in addressing trauma. In her sessions, she tapped on the various points while focusing on the car accident and the emotions associated with it. She used statements like, "Even though I feel terrified and helpless from the accident, I am ready to release this fear and pain."

As Sophia continued with EFT, she began to notice a shift in her emotional response to the traumatic memory. Her nightmares became less frequent, and when she did experience them, they were less intense. With continued tapping, Sophia found that her anxiety and fear around the accident gradually dissipated. EFT not only helped her manage PTSD symptoms but also empowered her to process and heal from the trauma in a way that traditional therapies had not.

Personal Story: Stress Reduction and Emotional Healing

Tina, a 38-year-old mother of two, had been experiencing overwhelming stress due to her demanding job and family obligations. She often felt exhausted, irritable, and disconnected from her emotions. Tina was recommended EFT by a friend and decided to give it a try.

In her first EFT session, Tina focused on the source of her stress—balancing work, family, and personal life. As she tapped on the acupressure points, she voiced statements like, "Even though I feel overwhelmed and stretched thin, I give myself permission to relax and take care of myself." The combination of the tapping process and the affirmations allowed Tina to process the emotions tied to her stress.

After several sessions, Tina noticed a significant reduction in her stress levels. She felt more in control of her emotions and was able to set clearer boundaries at work and at home. She also found that she could manage the demands of daily life with more patience and energy. This personal success story demonstrates how EFT can help individuals navigate stress and emotional overload, leading to greater emotional balance and resilience.

Case Study 4: Tackling Weight Loss and Emotional Eating

EFT has also been used effectively in the realm of emotional eating and weight loss. Mark, a 40-year-old man, struggled with his weight due to emotional eating. Whenever he felt stressed or anxious, he would reach for comfort food. His weight fluctuated, and he felt trapped in a cycle of emotional eating and self-blame.

Mark decided to try EFT to address the emotional triggers behind his eating habits. In his sessions, he focused on feelings of insecurity, stress, and the belief that food was a source of comfort. As he tapped on the acupressure points, Mark repeated affirmations such as, "Even though I turn to food for comfort when I'm stressed, I am learning to cope in healthier ways."

Over the course of several weeks, Mark noticed a shift in his relationship with food. He became more aware of his emotional triggers and was able to break the cycle of emotional eating. While his weight loss was gradual, the emotional healing he experienced through EFT was profound. Mark felt more in control of his actions, and his overall well-being improved.

The success stories and case studies surrounding EFT highlight its versatility and effectiveness as a therapeutic tool for addressing a wide range of emotional, psychological, and physical issues. From chronic pain and anxiety to trauma recovery and emotional eating, individuals have found relief through the combination of acupressure and emotional processing. Whether used in conjunction with other therapies or as a standalone practice, EFT provides a powerful way to release emotional blocks, reduce stress, and promote healing.

These personal experiences demonstrate that EFT is not just a quick fix but a tool for long-term emotional and physical well-being. As more people share their success stories, the growing body of evidence supporting EFT continues to inspire those seeking holistic approaches to healing and self-care.

As practitioners become more familiar with Emotional Freedom Technique (EFT), many choose to explore advanced practices that deepen the effectiveness of the method. While the basic EFT technique of tapping on specific acupressure points while voicing affirmations is highly effective for many, advanced EFT practices allow for more nuanced approaches, addressing deeper emotional issues, complex trauma, and multi-layered psychological challenges. These practices build on the foundational principles of EFT, enhancing its therapeutic benefits for those who are ready to explore more specialized techniques.

1. Matrix Reimprinting

Matrix Reimprinting is an advanced EFT technique that involves tapping on the body's energy system while also visualizing past traumatic memories or emotional blocks. Developed by Carl Dawson, Matrix Reimprinting takes EFT a step further by guiding individuals to revisit their memories and "reimprint" those experiences with more positive, healing emotions.

The process involves visualizing the younger version of yourself or the "traumatized part" of you in the memory. Through tapping, you work to transform the emotions tied to the memory, offering a new perspective and releasing old trauma patterns. The key idea behind Matrix Reimprinting is that the body retains emotional energy from past traumatic experiences, and by reimprinting those memories with new, healing energy, you can release the emotional charge tied to them.

This technique is particularly useful for individuals with deep-rooted trauma, such as abuse or childhood wounds, as it helps to change the energetic imprint of those memories and shift the emotional response tied to them.

2. Tailored Tapping Scripts

Advanced practitioners often tailor their tapping scripts to address more specific or complex issues. Instead of general statements like "Even though I have this pain, I deeply and completely accept myself," a more personalized script might target the unique aspects of a client's issue.

For instance, if someone is dealing with the fear of public speaking, a customized script may tap into the specific memories and fears associated with speaking in front of others, such as the feeling of judgment, past failures, or perceived inadequacies. The advanced practitioner will guide the client to focus on these specific emotional triggers while tapping through the points.

Personalized tapping scripts are an effective way to address issues that require a deeper, more targeted approach. These scripts help to ensure that the EFT session addresses all the layers of the problem, from conscious thoughts to subconscious beliefs.

3. Using EFT for Limiting Beliefs

Many people carry limiting beliefs that prevent them from achieving their goals or living fulfilling lives. These beliefs are often rooted in past experiences, childhood conditioning, or societal influences. In advanced EFT practices, practitioners use tapping to identify and shift these limiting beliefs by exploring their origins and replacing them with more empowering thoughts.

For example, a person who believes they are "not good enough" might have this belief linked to an early childhood experience. By tapping on the specific memory or emotion associated with that belief, they can release the energetic charge and shift their mindset. Over time, this practice can lead to greater self-confidence and personal empowerment.

4. EFT for Core Issues and Subconscious Blocks

Advanced EFT practitioners often work with clients to identify and release core issues or subconscious blocks that affect their behavior and emotional responses. Core issues are the fundamental beliefs or emotional wounds that tend to influence many areas of a person's life. For example, a core issue could be feelings of unworthiness, which might manifest in multiple ways—such as in relationships, career, or health.

By using advanced EFT, clients can identify these core issues through a process called "core belief excavation." This involves delving into a person's life history and discovering the root cause of recurring problems. Once the core issue is identified, EFT is used to address it directly, helping the individual release the emotional charge tied to the belief.

This practice often involves tapping through multiple layers of emotion and belief, as a single event or memory may be connected to a number of subconscious blocks. Through persistence and precision, advanced EFT can help individuals shift long-standing patterns of thinking and behavior.

5. EFT for Physical Conditions

While EFT is often used for emotional and psychological issues, advanced practitioners sometimes apply the technique to chronic or acute physical conditions. The belief is that physical pain or illness may have an emotional component that contributes to or exacerbates the condition. In advanced EFT, the practitioner will work with the client to identify any emotional trauma or stress that could be contributing to their physical symptoms.

For instance, if a person is dealing with chronic back pain, the practitioner may ask the client to reflect on any emotional triggers related to their back pain—such as feelings of burden, stress, or fear. By tapping on those emotional triggers, the body's energy system is recalibrated, often leading to a reduction in physical discomfort.

Advanced practitioners may also incorporate other modalities, such as guided imagery, affirmations, or neuro-linguistic programming (NLP), to help the individual release physical pain tied to emotional stress.

6. Advanced Emotional Release Techniques

In advanced EFT, practitioners may focus on deeper emotional release techniques that help clients let go of repressed emotions. Repressed emotions are feelings that are buried deep in the subconscious and often go unrecognized by the individual. These emotions may include anger, sadness, fear, or guilt that were suppressed due to societal pressures, childhood trauma, or other reasons.

Advanced EFT practitioners guide clients through a process of identifying these repressed emotions and tapping on them directly. By bringing these emotions into conscious awareness and releasing the emotional charge, individuals can experience a deep sense of relief and healing.

7. EFT and Energy Psychology

Energy psychology is an umbrella term for various therapeutic techniques that use the body's energy system to address emotional and physical health. Advanced EFT is often seen as a part of the broader field of energy psychology. Energy psychology techniques, such as Thought Field Therapy (TFT) or Psych-K, incorporate the same principles as EFT, focusing on the body's energy system to restore balance.

Advanced EFT practitioners may use techniques from these other modalities to complement traditional EFT tapping, offering clients a more holistic approach to healing. These practices can be especially useful for individuals dealing with trauma, phobias, or deeply ingrained patterns of behavior.

8. EFT and Spiritual Healing

In some advanced EFT practices, practitioners integrate spiritual or metaphysical elements into their sessions. This might involve tapping while focusing on concepts such as self-love, forgiveness, or spiritual growth. EFT is sometimes used to clear energetic blocks that are preventing the client from connecting with their higher self, manifesting their desires, or experiencing a sense of spiritual peace.

This approach may involve tapping on specific points while using spiritual affirmations or visualization techniques, such as imagining a healing light clearing the body's energy pathways. Spiritual EFT is often used by those seeking a more holistic form of healing that combines emotional, physical, and spiritual growth.

Advanced EFT practices offer a range of techniques designed to address deeper emotional, psychological, and physical issues. From Matrix Reimprinting and tailored tapping scripts to exploring core beliefs and subconscious blocks, these advanced methods allow practitioners to work with complex emotional layers and promote lasting change. Whether used to overcome trauma, heal from physical pain, or release limiting beliefs, advanced EFT practices provide powerful tools for healing and personal growth.

Advanced techniques and sequences in Emotional Freedom Technique (EFT) offer a more refined approach to addressing complex emotional issues, trauma, and chronic conditions. While the basic EFT sequence involves tapping on specific acupressure points while voicing affirmations, advanced methods go deeper by incorporating additional techniques, personalized tapping sequences, and addressing more intricate emotional layers. These advanced practices provide more effective and precise results for clients seeking deeper healing and transformation.

1. The Full Set of Points

The basic EFT tapping sequence uses a standard set of acupressure points. However, advanced practitioners often expand on this sequence to target additional points that can enhance the effectiveness of the technique. For example, tapping on points like the "gamut point" (located on the back of the hand) or using extra points on the body can address more complex issues or provide deeper emotional relief.

Advanced EFT practitioners may also experiment with tapping on the "small intestine" or "spleen" meridian points, which are linked to emotional regulation and stress management. This extended set of tapping points can be particularly useful when dealing with chronic stress, deep emotional wounds, or when more profound healing is needed.

2. Chasing the Pain

"Chasing the pain" is an advanced EFT strategy where practitioners continue to tap on a particular issue until all associated emotional discomfort dissipates. When clients experience pain or emotional discomfort, they are encouraged to focus on the sensation while tapping through the points.

In more advanced sequences, the practitioner helps the client track any changes in the sensation as they tap, guiding them to follow any shifts in the pain or emotion. For example, if a person is experiencing anxiety and feels a tightness in their chest, the practitioner may direct them to focus on the sensation in the chest and follow any changes that occur as they tap. This technique allows clients to address subtle shifts and uncover deeper emotional roots behind the pain or anxiety.

3. Advanced Voice and Words

Advanced EFT often incorporates more specific and personalized language to enhance emotional release. Rather than general statements like, "Even though I have this issue, I accept myself," advanced practitioners guide clients to tap with more focused and specific words, tailored to their individual experience.

For example, instead of simply saying, "Even though I feel stressed," an advanced sequence might include something like, "Even though I feel overwhelmed by my responsibilities and fear I'm not doing enough, I accept myself fully." By using more precise language, practitioners can help clients target the root cause of their emotional response and clear the emotional charge associated with it.

Furthermore, advanced practitioners may teach clients how to adjust their own tapping phrases during the session. As clients begin to identify new thoughts or feelings during the process, they can adapt their affirmations, leading to a more dynamic and effective release.

4. The Movie Technique

The "movie technique" is an advanced EFT approach used primarily for trauma or distressing memories. The client is guided to mentally replay a traumatic event or distressing situation, but instead of becoming overwhelmed by the emotions, they tap on the acupressure points while visualizing the memory. The process is much like watching a movie of the event, where the client distances themselves from the emotions attached to the memory.

During this technique, the practitioner helps the client keep the emotional intensity manageable by guiding them through the tapping sequence while they visualize the event in a neutral or detached way. The movie technique can help individuals reframe and release the emotional charge associated with traumatic experiences, often leading to a dramatic shift in their perception of the memory.

5. Tapping on Core Beliefs

Core beliefs are the deeply ingrained beliefs that people hold about themselves, others, and the world. These beliefs are often unconscious but have a significant impact on behavior and emotional well-being. Advanced EFT involves identifying and tapping on these core beliefs, especially those that are negative or limiting.

For example, if a person believes, "I am not good enough," advanced EFT might help them tap through the points while focusing on the origins of that belief, often tracing it back to childhood or pivotal life experiences. The practitioner will also help the client reframe these beliefs into more empowering statements, such as, "I am worthy of success and love." Releasing these core beliefs can be incredibly transformative, as they often influence multiple areas of a person's life, from relationships to career and personal well-being.

6. Releasing Emotions through the "Set-Up" Phase

The "set-up" phase in basic EFT involves identifying the issue and stating an affirmation that acknowledges both the problem and self-acceptance. In advanced EFT, however, practitioners may use this phase to dig deeper into the emotional layers connected to the issue. The goal is to identify the underlying emotions and limiting beliefs that may have been suppressed or ignored.

For example, during the set-up phase, a client may express an issue like, "I feel anxious about my job," but an advanced practitioner may explore deeper layers, like, "I fear rejection from my colleagues" or "I don't feel competent in my work." By tapping through these specific layers during the set-up, clients are able to target and release more nuanced emotions, creating a deeper sense of emotional freedom.

7. The "SUDs" Scale and Targeted Tapping

In EFT, the Subjective Units of Disturbance (SUDs) scale is used to measure the intensity of the emotional discomfort a client feels, with 10 being the highest level of discomfort and 0 being no discomfort at all. Advanced practitioners use this scale to help the client assess the intensity of their emotions and monitor progress throughout the tapping session.

Once a practitioner understands the client's emotional intensity, they can tailor the tapping sequence and adjust their approach based on the changes in the SUDs scale. If a client's SUDs score decreases during a session, the practitioner may continue tapping on specific emotions, beliefs, or memories to further reduce the emotional charge. This allows the practitioner to create a more effective and individualized treatment plan, ensuring that the client's specific issues are addressed and healed at the deepest level.

8. Tapping on the "Gamut Point"

The "gamut point," located on the back of the hand between the pinky and ring finger, is another advanced technique used in EFT. This point is associated with the regulation of brainwave patterns and is often included in advanced sequences to help shift the client's emotional state more quickly. During this step, the client taps the gamut point while simultaneously performing simple eye movements, humming, or counting aloud.

The gamut point helps to facilitate emotional release and can quickly shift brainwave states, making it particularly useful for rapid emotional regulation or when dealing with deeply entrenched emotional patterns. Practitioners may incorporate this point into the tapping sequence when they want to deepen the emotional release or enhance the clarity of thought and focus.

Advanced EFT techniques and sequences provide powerful tools for addressing deeper emotional wounds, chronic conditions, and complex trauma. From the movie technique and tapping on core beliefs to customized sequences and the gamut point, these advanced practices allow for a more nuanced approach to emotional healing. Whether you're addressing long-standing issues or working through more subtle emotional layers, these advanced techniques can help bring profound shifts and lasting relief. By deepening the EFT process, practitioners and clients can achieve greater emotional freedom, mental clarity, and physical healing.

Emotional Freedom Technique (EFT) is primarily known for its ability to address emotional, psychological, and physical issues, but its applications extend beyond these domains, including spiritual growth and personal transformation. While traditional spiritual practices focus on connecting to a higher self, cultivating inner peace, or deepening one's understanding of life's purpose, EFT can serve as a powerful tool to enhance this journey. By clearing emotional blockages and aligning the energy system, EFT allows individuals to move past limiting beliefs, fears, and patterns that hinder spiritual growth, facilitating deeper insights and a stronger connection to their spiritual path.

1. Clearing Emotional Blockages and Limiting Beliefs

One of the primary ways EFT supports spiritual growth is by clearing emotional blockages and limiting beliefs that may be preventing individuals from fully connecting with their spiritual self. Many people unknowingly carry beliefs that inhibit their spiritual development, such as feelings of unworthiness, fear of failure, or doubts about their connection to the universe. These negative beliefs can create resistance, keeping people stuck in patterns that prevent them from achieving a state of higher consciousness or spiritual clarity.

By using EFT to tap on the meridian points while voicing affirmations that challenge these limiting beliefs, individuals can release these blocks. For example, tapping on thoughts like, "Even though I feel unworthy of spiritual enlightenment, I accept myself completely," helps to shift the belief system and create space for a deeper spiritual connection. Over time, this emotional release creates a greater sense of openness, allowing the individual to embrace their spiritual journey without self-imposed limits.

2. Transforming Fear and Anxiety Around Spirituality

Fear and anxiety often arise when people are faced with spiritual challenges or new experiences on their path. This could include fear of the unknown, fear of spiritual failure, or anxiety about making significant life changes to align with one's higher purpose. EFT can be particularly useful in addressing these emotions by tapping into the root causes of fear and anxiety, often linked to past experiences or unresolved trauma.

For instance, a person might fear exploring new spiritual practices, such as meditation or yoga, because they associate them with past failures or feelings of inadequacy. By using EFT to tap on these specific fears, individuals can reframe their responses, reducing the emotional intensity and allowing them to approach spiritual growth with greater confidence and peace.

3. Enhancing Mindfulness and Self-Awareness

Spiritual growth requires a high degree of mindfulness and self-awareness. EFT can help individuals become more attuned to their emotions and thought patterns, facilitating a deeper understanding of their inner world. By regularly practicing EFT, individuals can identify and release unconscious beliefs or patterns that cloud their self-awareness. This heightened awareness can then be applied to their spiritual practice, leading to greater clarity and insight.

Through tapping, a person may uncover deeply held emotions or subconscious beliefs that were previously unacknowledged. These realizations help to clear mental clutter, fostering a deeper connection to one's authentic self and the present moment. As emotional blockages dissolve, individuals can move into a state of greater clarity and awareness, enhancing their ability to engage in spiritual practices like meditation, prayer, or contemplation.

4. Releasing Emotional Trauma for Healing and Growth

Emotional trauma, whether from childhood experiences, relationships, or past life experiences, can significantly affect one's ability to grow spiritually. Trauma often leads to a distorted sense of self or a disconnect from one's true nature. EFT is highly effective in helping individuals process and release emotional trauma stored in the body's energy system.

By tapping on the specific acupressure points while focusing on traumatic memories or emotional wounds, EFT facilitates the release of stored emotional energy, allowing for healing and spiritual growth. This healing process can create a sense of emotional freedom and open up space for a more authentic spiritual connection. Once past traumas are cleared, individuals may experience greater emotional balance, clarity of thought, and an ability to align with their spiritual goals.

5. Aligning with Higher Purpose

As individuals progress on their spiritual journey, they often seek to align more deeply with their higher purpose or life mission. However, the presence of unresolved emotions or limiting beliefs can make this alignment difficult. EFT helps to clear these mental and emotional barriers, enabling individuals to tap into their intuition and connect with their true calling.

For example, someone may feel disconnected from their sense of purpose because they hold subconscious beliefs about their inability to succeed or their unworthiness of a meaningful life. EFT allows them to tap through these beliefs, creating a more open channel for clarity and insight. This process can help individuals feel more aligned with their higher self and the divine plan, allowing them to move forward with greater confidence and a sense of spiritual direction.

6. Cultivating Compassion and Self-Love

A key element of spiritual growth is the cultivation of compassion, both for oneself and others. EFT is particularly effective in fostering self-love by addressing negative self-talk, guilt, or self-judgment, which can prevent individuals from feeling deserving of love and compassion. By tapping on these emotions, people can release feelings of inadequacy or unworthiness and replace them with self-compassion and acceptance.

For instance, someone who struggles with feelings of guilt for past mistakes can use EFT to release the emotional charge associated with those feelings. Tapping through the points while focusing on affirmations like, "Even though I feel guilty about past actions, I forgive myself and choose to love myself," can help to shift the emotional state. Over time, this practice enhances self-love, creating a stronger foundation for spiritual growth and connection.

7. Accessing a Higher State of Consciousness

EFT can also be used to facilitate a higher state of consciousness, which is a critical aspect of spiritual growth. As individuals release emotional baggage and limiting beliefs, they often experience a sense of expanded awareness or a shift in consciousness. This state of heightened awareness opens the door for greater spiritual insights, intuitive guidance, and deep personal transformation.

By clearing emotional blockages, EFT practitioners can access a state of "flow" where spiritual experiences or insights can naturally arise. This practice can enhance spiritual practices such as meditation, prayer, or journaling, as it allows individuals to experience greater peace, clarity, and openness to receiving spiritual guidance.

8. EFT for Chakras and Energy Centers

In addition to working on emotional and psychological blockages, EFT can be used to clear blockages in the body's energy centers, such as the chakras. Each chakra is associated with different emotional, mental, and spiritual aspects of a person's life. When a chakra is blocked, it can affect physical health, emotional well-being, and spiritual alignment.

By focusing on specific chakras and tapping through the EFT sequence while concentrating on the energy flow in each center, individuals can release energetic blockages and bring their chakras into balance. For example, tapping while focusing on the heart chakra can help release feelings of grief or unresolved emotional pain, opening the heart to more love and compassion. This process can significantly enhance spiritual practices, as it creates greater energetic alignment and balance within the body.

EFT is a versatile and effective tool for enhancing spiritual growth, providing individuals with the ability to release emotional blockages, overcome limiting beliefs, and deepen their connection to their higher self. By addressing the emotional, mental, and energetic components of spiritual development, EFT clears the path for greater awareness, self-love, and alignment with one's true purpose. Whether used to heal past trauma, cultivate compassion, or achieve a higher state of consciousness, EFT offers profound benefits for those seeking to enhance their spiritual journey.

Many individuals have experienced profound transformations through advanced EFT practices, where the technique is applied to complex issues like trauma, chronic pain, limiting beliefs, and spiritual growth. These success stories highlight the power of EFT to not only heal emotional wounds but also enhance personal development and overall well-being.

1. Overcoming Childhood Trauma

A woman in her 40s, who had experienced severe emotional trauma as a child, used advanced EFT techniques to work through her deeply rooted fears and anxieties. Despite years of traditional therapy, she found herself stuck in recurring patterns of self-doubt and fear, especially when it came to trusting others. Through advanced EFT, she used techniques like the "movie technique" to tap on past traumatic memories while staying emotionally detached from them. As she progressed, she noticed a significant shift in her ability to trust others and in her general emotional stability. Over several sessions, she reported feeling lighter, more confident, and capable of maintaining healthier relationships, which had previously been a challenge.

2. Chronic Pain Relief

A man suffering from chronic back pain for over 10 years sought relief using advanced EFT. His pain was not only physical but was also tied to unresolved emotional issues stemming from a past accident. Traditional treatments had provided temporary relief, but the pain would always return. Using the "chasing the pain" technique, where the practitioner helped him focus on the pain while tapping through the meridian points, he was able to trace the emotional components tied to the physical discomfort. By addressing the emotional trauma connected to the injury and tapping on it, he experienced a remarkable reduction in pain and, for the first time in years, was able to perform daily activities without discomfort.

3. Release of Limiting Beliefs

A man in his 30s, frustrated with his career stagnation, turned to advanced EFT to address limiting beliefs around his ability to succeed. He had always felt that he wasn't worthy of promotions or opportunities, often sabotaging his own progress. Through tapping on specific meridian points and focusing on his deep-rooted beliefs like "I am not good enough" and "I will never be successful," he was able to release these beliefs. With the help of tailored affirmations during his sessions, he reframed these thoughts into empowering statements. Within a few weeks, he not only gained a new sense of confidence but also landed a promotion he had long desired, which he attributes to the emotional clearing that EFT provided.

4. Resolving Relationship Issues

A couple dealing with chronic relationship conflicts used advanced EFT to address the underlying emotional issues that were causing their repeated arguments and disconnect. They each had different emotional triggers and unresolved past experiences that would resurface in their interactions. With advanced EFT, they worked through these triggers by identifying core beliefs and tapping on specific emotional reactions. One key breakthrough involved addressing unspoken resentment that had built up over the years. After several sessions, both reported feeling more empathetic towards each other, with improved communication and a stronger emotional bond.

5. Emotional and Spiritual Alignment

A woman who had been practicing spirituality for many years but felt disconnected and stagnant sought EFT for deeper emotional and spiritual alignment. She struggled with feelings of unworthiness and self-doubt, which kept her from fully embracing her spiritual practices. By using advanced tapping techniques to clear these emotional blocks, particularly tapping on the heart chakra and focusing on self-love and forgiveness, she found a renewed sense of purpose. Within a few months, her meditation practice deepened, and she began receiving clearer insights during her sessions. She reported feeling more connected to her higher self and experienced a significant spiritual breakthrough, feeling more at peace and aligned with her true purpose.

6. Coping with Anxiety and Public Speaking Fear

A client who had struggled with severe anxiety around public speaking for years used advanced EFT to reduce the emotional charge attached to her fear. She had tried various methods without success, but advanced tapping allowed her to dive deeper into the root causes of her fear—mainly, past traumatic experiences of being ridiculed in front of groups. Using the "movie technique," she was able to revisit these memories while tapping, diminishing the intensity of her anxiety. After several sessions, she confidently delivered a presentation to a large audience, something she had avoided for most of her life. The EFT sessions helped her release the anxiety tied to public speaking and enabled her to perform without fear.

7. Overcoming Addiction Triggers

An individual in recovery from alcohol addiction used advanced EFT to address the triggers and emotional patterns that led to relapse. Through tapping on specific emotional memories and beliefs around stress, self-worth, and past trauma, the individual found relief from the powerful cravings that once dominated their life. Using the "gamut point" technique, combined with focused tapping on the core emotional roots of addiction, they experienced a significant shift in their ability to manage triggers without resorting to alcohol. After consistent use of EFT, they maintained long-term sobriety and reported feeling more in control of their emotional responses and triggers.

These success stories demonstrate how advanced EFT can facilitate deep emotional healing and lead to lasting transformation in areas such as trauma, relationships, career, spiritual growth, and addiction recovery. The personalized nature of EFT, along with its ability to address both emotional and physical aspects of a problem, allows individuals to make profound shifts, empowering them to lead healthier, more fulfilling lives.

Emotional Freedom Technique (EFT) has emerged as a highly sought-after therapeutic method, gaining recognition among both mental health professionals and those seeking to enhance personal growth. As more individuals and organizations embrace EFT, the demand for qualified practitioners continues to rise, creating diverse career opportunities in the field. Pursuing certification in EFT not only provides an in-depth understanding of the technique but also opens the door to a variety of career paths.

1. What is EFT Certification?

EFT certification is a formal process by which individuals gain professional recognition for their knowledge and skill in applying Emotional Freedom Technique. Certification programs are offered by various organizations and typically require completing training courses, demonstrating proficiency in EFT practice, and often passing exams or assessments. These programs are designed to ensure that practitioners possess the necessary knowledge and ethical understanding to use EFT effectively and safely with clients.

Certified EFT practitioners learn to apply the technique to a wide range of issues, including emotional trauma, stress, anxiety, phobias, chronic pain, and more. The certification process also teaches practitioners how to customize EFT interventions for individual clients, making it a highly personalized and client-centered therapy.

2. Types of EFT Certifications

There are several types of EFT certifications, catering to different levels of expertise and specialization. Commonly recognized certification levels include:

- **Basic Certification:** This entry-level certification equips individuals with foundational knowledge of EFT. It covers the basics of tapping, the meridian system, and how to apply EFT to common emotional and physical issues.
- **Intermediate and Advanced Certification:** These certifications build on basic knowledge and teach more advanced techniques, such as working with deeper emotional issues, trauma, limiting beliefs, and chronic pain. Advanced practitioners learn specialized protocols for more complex client needs.
- **Master Certification:** Master-level certification is for those who want to deepen their expertise and become leaders in the EFT community. These programs usually focus on advanced interventions, research-based applications, and training other practitioners.

Many certification programs also offer specializations, such as EFT for trauma, children, relationships, or addictions, allowing practitioners to refine their skills in a niche area of practice.

3. Career Opportunities with EFT Certification

Obtaining EFT certification opens up a wide array of career opportunities. EFT practitioners can work in a variety of settings, providing therapeutic services, teaching, or consulting. Some common career paths for certified EFT practitioners include:

- **Private Practice:** Many EFT-certified professionals choose to open their own private practice, offering one-on-one sessions or group workshops. This career path provides flexibility and the ability to work with clients on a broad range of issues.
- **Therapists and Counselors:** EFT is increasingly integrated into traditional therapy practices, allowing licensed counselors, psychologists, and social workers to enhance their existing services. EFT is particularly valuable for therapists working with clients experiencing trauma, anxiety, phobias, and emotional distress.
- **Corporate Wellness Programs:** With increasing awareness of the importance of mental health, many companies are incorporating EFT into their employee wellness programs. Certified EFT practitioners can offer workshops or individual sessions to help employees manage stress, improve emotional well-being, and enhance productivity.
- **Life Coaches and Personal Development:** Certified EFT practitioners are well-suited to work as life coaches, helping individuals overcome personal obstacles, such as self-doubt, limiting beliefs, and past trauma. EFT can be a powerful tool for personal transformation, making it an attractive addition to the life coaching toolbox.
- **Addiction Recovery and Support:** EFT is widely used in addiction recovery to help individuals address emotional triggers, cravings, and past trauma. Certified

EFT practitioners may work in rehabilitation centers, support groups, or as part of a recovery team, helping clients release emotional blocks that contribute to addictive behaviors.
- **Workshops and Seminars:** Many certified EFT practitioners teach the technique to others through workshops and seminars, sharing their expertise and empowering individuals to use EFT for their own personal growth. These events can be hosted in person or online, allowing practitioners to reach a wider audience.
- **Training and Mentorship:** Experienced EFT practitioners with Master Certification can also take on a teaching or mentorship role, training the next generation of EFT professionals. These opportunities can involve creating educational materials, leading training programs, and mentoring new practitioners.

4. Benefits of EFT Certification

Becoming certified in EFT offers numerous benefits, including:

- **Credibility and Professional Recognition:** Certification lends credibility to practitioners, signaling to clients that they have met rigorous standards and are qualified to provide EFT therapy. It can also increase trust and confidence among potential clients.
- **Personal Growth and Development:** EFT certification programs often involve deep personal work as well as professional training. Practitioners may experience significant personal growth as they apply EFT to their own lives, improving their emotional well-being and gaining firsthand experience of the technique's effectiveness.
- **Increased Client Success:** A certified EFT practitioner is more likely to achieve successful outcomes with clients because they have been trained in a range of techniques and understand how to tailor EFT interventions to meet individual needs. Clients benefit from working with a practitioner who has expertise and knowledge of best practices.
- **Networking and Community Support:** EFT certification connects practitioners to a global community of like-minded individuals, offering networking opportunities, peer support, and continued professional development. This community can be an invaluable resource for ongoing learning and collaboration.
- **Flexibility and Independence:** Certification in EFT allows practitioners to design their own careers, whether through private practice, corporate work, or educational roles. The ability to work remotely or set flexible hours is an attractive aspect for many EFT professionals.

5. How to Get Started

Becoming a certified EFT practitioner typically involves the following steps:

1. **Find a Reputable Certification Program:** Research organizations that offer EFT certification, such as the EFT International (EFTi) or The EFT Academy. Look for a program that is accredited and recognized within the EFT community.
2. **Complete Training and Coursework:** Enroll in the chosen EFT program, which may include online courses, in-person workshops, and practical assignments. The training will cover both theoretical knowledge and practical application.
3. **Practice and Apply EFT:** Most certification programs require a certain number of hours of practice, either through self-application or by working with clients under supervision. This helps to develop proficiency and confidence in the technique.
4. **Pass the Certification Exam:** Many programs require an exam or assessment to demonstrate mastery of EFT. This could include written exams, case studies, or live demonstrations of tapping techniques.
5. **Stay Updated and Engage in Continuous Learning:** To maintain certification, many EFT organizations require practitioners to continue their education, attend workshops, and engage in professional development activities.

EFT certification provides a powerful opportunity for individuals to embark on a rewarding career as an emotional wellness professional. Whether working in private practice, corporate wellness, addiction recovery, or as a life coach, certified EFT practitioners are able to offer effective, personalized interventions that help clients achieve lasting emotional freedom. With an increasing demand for alternative therapies, EFT is a promising field for those passionate about helping others heal, grow, and thrive.

The process of becoming an EFT practitioner

Becoming an EFT practitioner involves a structured process that equips individuals with the skills, knowledge, and confidence to effectively apply Emotional Freedom Technique with clients. The path to certification is designed to ensure practitioners can use EFT safely, ethically, and proficiently, allowing them to offer support to individuals dealing with emotional, physical, or psychological challenges.

1. Initial Training and Education

The first step in becoming an EFT practitioner is to enroll in a comprehensive EFT training program. There are numerous organizations that offer accredited EFT certification courses, each with its own approach but generally following core principles of EFT. The training typically covers the fundamentals of EFT, including the theory behind the technique, the meridian system, and how emotions are processed in the body.

Training programs usually begin with a foundational course, often referred to as Level 1, which introduces students to the basic tapping points and teaches them how to perform EFT on themselves. Level 1 focuses on self-application and allows students to experience firsthand how the technique works for emotional release and healing. This personal experience is crucial for practitioners as it builds their understanding of EFT's effectiveness and empowers them to share it with others.

2. Understanding the Core Concepts of EFT

Before becoming a certified practitioner, it's important to have a solid understanding of the core principles that guide EFT. These include:

- **The Meridian System:** The technique is based on the idea that the body's energy system is connected to physical and emotional health. EFT uses tapping on specific acupressure points along the body's meridians to release blocked energy and promote emotional balance.
- **The Mind-Body Connection:** EFT operates under the principle that emotional distress and trauma can manifest physically, and addressing these emotions can lead to improvements in both mental and physical well-being. Practitioners must

understand how deeply emotions are connected to physical sensations and symptoms.
- **The Role of Emotional Blocks:** EFT helps practitioners identify and work through emotional blocks that may be causing pain, stress, or other psychological issues. These blocks are believed to stem from unresolved past experiences, limiting beliefs, or trauma.

3. Practical Application and Supervised Practice

Once you've completed the introductory training, the next step involves hands-on practice. This is essential for building competence and confidence. In many certification programs, students are required to practice EFT on themselves, friends, or family members, and then submit case studies or reflections on the sessions. Some programs also offer supervised practice, where students work directly with clients under the guidance of an experienced EFT instructor.

Practical sessions help aspiring practitioners refine their technique, develop a personalized tapping style, and understand how to handle different emotional situations that may arise in a client session. Supervised practice ensures that students receive feedback, which helps them improve their skills and ensure they are using EFT ethically and effectively.

4. Advanced EFT Training

After mastering the basic level, aspiring practitioners often proceed to more advanced training. Level 2 and Level 3 courses dive deeper into specific techniques, such as working with trauma, addictions, limiting beliefs, and complex emotional issues. These advanced programs teach practitioners how to apply EFT to deeper emotional and physical challenges, customize interventions for individual clients, and address more nuanced issues that may arise during sessions.

Advanced courses also teach more sophisticated techniques such as the "movie technique," "choices method," and working with the inner child or parts therapy. The ability to utilize these specialized techniques makes practitioners more effective when dealing with complex client issues and ensures they can deliver a broad range of interventions based on the individual needs of each client.

5. Certification Requirements and Exam

After completing the required training and supervised practice hours, most certification programs require candidates to demonstrate their proficiency in EFT. Certification exams may include practical assessments, written tests, or the submission of case studies that show the applicant's ability to effectively use EFT in real-world situations.

The examination process ensures that EFT practitioners have a comprehensive understanding of the technique and can apply it ethically and safely in a therapeutic setting. Successful completion of the exam and submission of required materials generally leads to certification.

6. Ongoing Professional Development

EFT certification is not a one-time achievement. Practitioners are encouraged to continue their education and develop their skills over time. Many certification programs require continuing education credits to maintain certification. These ongoing learning opportunities may include advanced workshops, conferences, and specialized courses in areas such as trauma recovery, stress management, or EFT for children.

Regular participation in professional development activities ensures that practitioners stay updated on new techniques, research, and best practices in EFT. It also helps them remain active in the EFT community and stay connected with other professionals.

7. Ethical and Professional Guidelines

An important part of becoming an EFT practitioner involves understanding and adhering to ethical standards and professional guidelines. EFT practitioners are expected to operate within a framework that prioritizes the well-being and safety of clients. This includes maintaining confidentiality, obtaining informed consent, and referring clients to other professionals when necessary.

Ethical guidelines also emphasize the importance of using EFT responsibly, ensuring that it is applied in a way that benefits the client and avoids any harm. Practitioners must also understand the limitations of their role and seek supervision or further training when dealing with more complex or serious mental health issues.

8. Setting Up a Practice

Once certified, EFT practitioners can begin working with clients. Some may choose to establish a private practice, while others may work in existing therapy clinics, wellness centers, or corporate environments. In addition to offering one-on-one EFT sessions, practitioners may choose to lead group workshops, teach classes, or offer online services.

Marketing and business management are also key elements of establishing a successful practice. EFT practitioners often need to develop skills in client acquisition, social media marketing, and professional networking to attract clients and grow their practice.

Becoming an EFT practitioner involves a combination of formal training, practical experience, and continuous professional development. The process empowers individuals to support others in overcoming emotional challenges and achieving greater well-being. By learning both the technical and interpersonal aspects of EFT, practitioners are equipped to offer profound healing and transformation to those seeking emotional freedom. Whether working in private practice, corporate settings, or as part of a healthcare team, certified EFT practitioners can make a lasting impact on their clients' lives.

Types of EFT therapy careers

A career in Emotional Freedom Technique (EFT) offers a broad range of opportunities for those interested in helping others achieve emotional well-being. EFT practitioners work across various sectors, from private practice to corporate wellness programs, offering support for a diverse array of issues, such as stress, anxiety, trauma, and chronic pain. The flexibility and versatility of EFT allow professionals to carve out niche careers or work in collaborative environments alongside other therapists, coaches, or health professionals.

1. Private Practice EFT Practitioner

One of the most common career paths for certified EFT practitioners is to open a private practice. This allows practitioners to work one-on-one with clients, offering personalized sessions tailored to the individual's needs. Private practice provides flexibility in terms of working hours and client base. Practitioners can offer services in-person or online, making it easier to reach clients from various geographical locations.

Clients seeking EFT in a private practice setting may be dealing with emotional trauma, stress, anxiety, phobias, limiting beliefs, or physical pain. EFT practitioners in private practice often work with individuals, couples, or families to help them overcome emotional blocks, process past trauma, and achieve personal growth.

2. Corporate Wellness and Stress Management Specialist

With an increasing focus on employee well-being, many companies are integrating EFT into their corporate wellness programs. This role involves using EFT to help employees manage stress, reduce anxiety, and improve overall emotional health. EFT can be applied in workshops, seminars, or one-on-one sessions to address work-related stressors, burnout, or personal issues that affect productivity and well-being.

Corporate wellness EFT practitioners often collaborate with human resources departments, organizational psychologists, and wellness consultants to design customized programs that promote a positive work culture. As workplace stress continues to be a major concern for employers, professionals trained in EFT are increasingly sought after in this field.

3. EFT and Mental Health Therapy

Many licensed therapists and counselors incorporate EFT into their existing therapeutic practices. By adding EFT to their toolkit, mental health professionals can offer an alternative to traditional talk therapy, especially for clients dealing with unresolved emotional trauma, anxiety, depression, or phobias. EFT provides an additional layer of support, especially when clients are struggling to make progress with conventional methods.

In this role, EFT practitioners often work alongside other therapeutic modalities such as cognitive-behavioral therapy (CBT), mindfulness, or psychodynamic therapy. The integration of EFT allows therapists to target the emotional and energetic components of a client's struggles, leading to faster and more lasting results.

4. Life Coach or Personal Development Practitioner

Life coaches trained in EFT use the technique to help clients overcome personal obstacles, limiting beliefs, and emotional challenges that may be hindering their progress. EFT provides a powerful tool for clients who want to achieve specific goals, whether related to career advancement, personal growth, or relationship improvement.

EFT coaches can work with clients on a variety of issues, including self-confidence, motivation, stress management, or achieving work-life balance. These professionals often use EFT as part of a broader coaching framework, combining it with other techniques like goal-setting, visualization, and accountability strategies.

5. EFT for Trauma and PTSD Specialist

EFT is widely recognized for its effectiveness in addressing trauma and post-traumatic stress disorder (PTSD). Practitioners specializing in trauma recovery use EFT to help individuals release emotional and psychological scars from past events, whether from childhood abuse, accidents, or military combat. EFT can be used to address both acute and long-standing trauma.

Professionals in this field often work with clients who have experienced severe emotional distress and need specialized interventions. By focusing on trauma at the emotional and energetic level, EFT allows clients to release long-held pain and begin the healing process.

Specializing in trauma and PTSD may require additional training and expertise, such as understanding the physiological and psychological aspects of trauma and its effects on the body and mind.

6. EFT for Addictions

Addiction recovery is another area where EFT practitioners can make a significant impact. EFT has proven to be highly effective in addressing the emotional and psychological components of addiction, helping clients reduce cravings, manage withdrawal symptoms, and heal underlying trauma that may contribute to addictive behaviors.

EFT for addiction may be used in conjunction with other therapeutic approaches such as cognitive-behavioral therapy (CBT) or 12-step programs. Practitioners in this field often work with individuals struggling with substance abuse, eating disorders, or behavioral addictions like gambling or compulsive behaviors.

In addition to one-on-one sessions, EFT practitioners may lead group sessions or workshops for addiction recovery, providing support in a more community-oriented setting.

7. EFT for Chronic Pain and Illness

Chronic pain and illness are often influenced by emotional and psychological factors. EFT practitioners specializing in pain management use the technique to help clients manage and alleviate symptoms associated with conditions like fibromyalgia, chronic back pain, migraines, and autoimmune disorders. EFT works by addressing the emotional triggers that may exacerbate pain, such as stress, unresolved emotions, or past trauma.

Many clients seeking EFT for chronic pain find that the emotional and energetic release provided by tapping can lead to noticeable improvements in physical symptoms. Practitioners in this field often work alongside medical professionals to provide complementary care.

8. EFT Trainer or Instructor

For those with extensive experience in EFT, becoming a trainer or instructor can be a rewarding career option. EFT trainers are responsible for educating new practitioners, teaching foundational and advanced EFT techniques, and offering certification programs. This role involves not only technical knowledge but also the ability to communicate complex concepts clearly and provide hands-on guidance to students.

EFT instructors may work with individuals or groups, either in-person or online, and often lead workshops, retreats, or continuing education programs. Successful trainers can also contribute to the broader EFT community by writing books, creating online courses, or speaking at conferences and events.

9. Group Facilitator

Group facilitation is another career path for EFT practitioners, especially those who prefer working with multiple people at once. Group EFT sessions are often used for addressing general emotional health, stress relief, or personal development. These group sessions can be highly effective in creating a sense of community and shared healing.

Facilitators may lead regular tapping groups, workshops, or themed events for specific issues such as anxiety, grief, or trauma recovery. Group EFT can provide a supportive environment for individuals to share their experiences while benefiting from the collective energy of the group.

10. EFT Researcher

For those interested in the academic side of EFT, pursuing a career as a researcher allows individuals to contribute to the growing body of evidence supporting EFT's effectiveness. EFT researchers often conduct studies to investigate its impact on various physical, emotional, and psychological conditions, and work in collaboration with universities, health institutions, or research organizations.

Research can focus on a variety of topics, such as the efficacy of EFT in treating PTSD, chronic pain, or anxiety, or the mechanisms behind how EFT works on the body's energy system. Publishing research results and collaborating with other scientists can help validate EFT as a mainstream therapeutic modality.

The versatility of EFT as a therapeutic technique creates numerous career opportunities for those passionate about helping others. Whether working in private practice, corporate wellness, trauma recovery, or addiction treatment, EFT practitioners can make a significant impact in improving emotional and physical health. With the right training and expertise, EFT professionals can choose from a wide range of career paths, allowing them to personalize their practice and create a meaningful, impactful career in the field of emotional wellness.

Emotional Freedom Technique tips

- Start by identifying the issue or emotion you want to address.
- Focus on how the emotion makes you feel in your body.
- Use the phrase "Even though I have this [feeling/emotion], I deeply and completely accept myself."
- Keep your statements specific to your emotional experience.
- Use neutral or positive language when phrasing affirmations.
- Tap on both sides of the body to enhance balance.
- Adjust the tapping pressure to your comfort.
- Tap with your fingertips, not your full hand.
- Don't skip the setup statement—it's crucial for emotional release.
- Use the "even though" phrase to acknowledge the emotion, without judgment.
- Make sure your setup statement feels true to you.
- Re-evaluate the emotional intensity after each round of tapping.
- Aim for a SUDS (Subjective Units of Distress) level of 0 after tapping.
- Avoid tapping on painful or broken areas of the body.
- If tapping doesn't feel effective, try reframing your statement.
- Remember, EFT works on both emotional and physical pain.
- Use your intuition to adapt your tapping sequence.
- Revisit previous trauma with patience and kindness.
- When working with trauma, tap gently and slowly.
- Pay attention to any shifts in physical sensations during tapping.
- Use positive affirmations once the intensity of the issue decreases.
- Tap on each acupressure point 5-7 times for best results.
- Tap on all the points, but don't worry about memorizing them perfectly.
- If a particular point causes discomfort, ease up on the tapping pressure.
- For deep emotional issues, break them into smaller components for more manageable sessions.
- Practice EFT daily for maximum emotional relief.
- Include gratitude statements during your tapping to shift your energy.
- Keep your phrasing flexible to match your emotional experience.
- For chronic issues, repeat the process consistently over time.
- Tap even if you're unsure if the issue is fully resolved—more layers may surface.
- When dealing with physical pain, tap on the pain area but not directly on a wound.
- Integrate EFT into your meditation practice for deeper relaxation.

- You can tap before or after other forms of therapy.
- Stay mindful of your breathing while tapping—it helps with relaxation.
- Be patient with your emotional healing process.
- If you experience resistance, try tapping on the resistance itself.
- Combine tapping with visualization techniques for deeper impact.
- Use EFT for performance anxiety or public speaking fear.
- Reframe negative beliefs with EFT to transform your mindset.
- Tap with a specific issue in mind, but be open to other emotions arising.
- Utilize the "tearless trauma technique" for dealing with intense memories.
- Check in with yourself regularly to assess emotional progress.
- Tap on limiting beliefs to unlock your full potential.
- Use EFT to release judgment and self-criticism.
- Apply EFT to increase self-confidence and self-love.
- Avoid rushing the tapping process—allow emotions to arise naturally.
- If you experience unexpected emotional releases, allow them to unfold.
- Tap on frustration or feelings of "stuckness" to regain clarity.
- Pair EFT with deep breathing exercises for relaxation.
- Use EFT for weight loss by tapping on emotional blocks to weight.
- When tapping on an intense emotion, focus on how it feels in your body.
- Tap with your eyes closed if it helps you to focus better.
- If a topic is too overwhelming, break it into smaller issues and tackle one at a time.
- Tap on financial worries or abundance blocks to improve financial health.
- Use EFT for relationship issues by tapping on emotional triggers or misunderstandings.
- Tap on areas where you feel physical discomfort alongside emotional issues.
- Combine EFT with journaling to clarify your emotions before tapping.
- Use tapping to alleviate sleep issues caused by overthinking or anxiety.
- Practice EFT on everyday stressors to prevent emotional buildup.
- Use tapping when dealing with past trauma that surfaces unexpectedly.
- If you're feeling overwhelmed, tap slowly and gently to calm your nervous system.
- Don't rush the process—slow, steady tapping is most effective.
- Focus on your present feelings rather than trying to solve everything at once.
- Tap through childhood memories if they're contributing to your current issues.
- Practice EFT to release old emotional wounds from relationships.
- Tap with specific symptoms, such as headaches or digestive issues, to find relief.
- Always acknowledge your emotional state before tapping.
- Tap on the feelings of guilt or shame to release them.
- When tapping on sadness, focus on any tightness or heaviness in your body.
- Tap on feelings of rejection or fear of failure to rewire your beliefs.
- Use tapping to build resilience and emotional strength.

- Tap on any feelings of fear related to future events or unknown outcomes.
- Practice EFT to reduce the intensity of emotional flashbacks.
- Tap for better decision-making when you feel indecisive or conflicted.
- Use EFT when experiencing feelings of overwhelm or burnout.
- When working with grief, tap on the pain of loss and emotional numbness.
- If your emotions feel "stuck," try tapping on the phrase "Even though I feel stuck..."
- Focus on how your emotions physically manifest in your body while tapping.
- Use EFT to clear emotional baggage from past mistakes or regrets.
- Incorporate tapping into your self-care routine for emotional balance.
- Tap for self-worth and to shift from self-doubt to self-assurance.
- Use EFT to release anger in a healthy and productive way.
- Be open to the possibility that EFT may take time to show results.
- For chronic issues, tap on both the physical symptoms and emotional triggers.
- Tap on feelings of helplessness to regain a sense of control.
- Use EFT to break old patterns and habits that no longer serve you.
- Tap for clarity when you feel confused or uncertain about a decision.
- Keep a log of your tapping progress to track emotional shifts.
- When tapping for anxiety, focus on the feeling of tension in your body.
- If you feel resistance, tap on the belief that it won't work.
- Use EFT to release negative thought patterns that hold you back.
- Tap on any unresolved emotions related to past traumas, big or small.
- Tap on the fear of not being good enough or imposter syndrome.
- Combine EFT with positive affirmations to increase its effectiveness.
- Tap on frustration when things aren't going as planned.
- Focus on relaxation when tapping for stress-related issues.
- Use EFT to overcome fear of change or fear of the unknown.
- Tap for personal empowerment and to remove feelings of powerlessness.
- Incorporate tapping into your routine to prevent emotional overwhelm.
- For health-related issues, tap to release stress and promote healing.
- Tap on old family patterns or generational issues that influence your current emotions.
- Release fears around success and the responsibilities that come with it.
- Tap on limiting beliefs regarding love and relationships.
- Use EFT to enhance creativity and release mental blocks.
- Tap to regain a sense of peace after an emotional upset.
- Use tapping to clear emotional resistance to success or prosperity.
- Tap to overcome procrastination by addressing underlying fears or beliefs.
- Tap on feelings of fear or uncertainty about the future.
- Use EFT to release feelings of loneliness or isolation.

- Tap for emotional balance when you're feeling overwhelmed by life's demands.
- Tap for clarity and direction when you're feeling lost or uncertain.
- Tap on anger that stems from feeling misunderstood or unheard.
- When you feel stuck in negative patterns, tap to shift your mindset.
- Tap for confidence when preparing for a challenging event or situation.
- Tap to release perfectionism and embrace self-compassion.
- Use EFT for energy clearing, removing emotional blockages from the body.
- Tap on physical discomfort caused by emotional strain, such as tight shoulders or headaches.
- Use tapping to release unhealthy attachments to people or situations.
- Focus on the physical sensation of fear when tapping on anxiety.
- Tap on feelings of inadequacy or self-criticism to increase self-acceptance.
- Use EFT to boost motivation when you feel discouraged.
- Tap to shift your energy from negative to positive states.
- Practice tapping daily to prevent emotional buildup from stress or anxiety.
- Use EFT for empowerment and to release feelings of victimhood.
- Tap on any unresolved conflict within your relationships.
- Tap to ease your emotions before major life transitions.
- Use tapping as a tool for self-love and acceptance.
- Tap on the fear of being judged or criticized by others.
- Tap on feelings of grief, loss, or unresolved sorrow.
- Use EFT to shift self-sabotaging patterns into productive behaviors.
- Tap to release guilt associated with past decisions or actions.
- Tap for personal growth and breaking through emotional barriers.
- If you feel overwhelmed by life's challenges, tap for resilience.
- Use EFT to break free from unhealthy patterns of dependence.
- Tap on fear of rejection or abandonment to feel more secure.
- Focus on the root of the issue when using EFT to achieve lasting results.
- Tap to increase feelings of peace and inner calm.
- Tap for grounding when you feel emotionally scattered.
- Tap on feelings of disconnection from your true self.
- Tap to release any lingering anxiety from past events.
- Use EFT to break emotional ties to negative experiences or people.
- Tap on fear of losing control or being vulnerable.
- Incorporate EFT to reduce fear of confrontation.
- Tap for emotional freedom after experiencing trauma or a setback.
- Use EFT to shift negative thinking patterns into constructive ones.
- Tap for clarity when you feel stuck in indecision or confusion.
- Tap on feelings of being overwhelmed by the demands of others.
- Use EFT to improve emotional resilience in difficult situations.

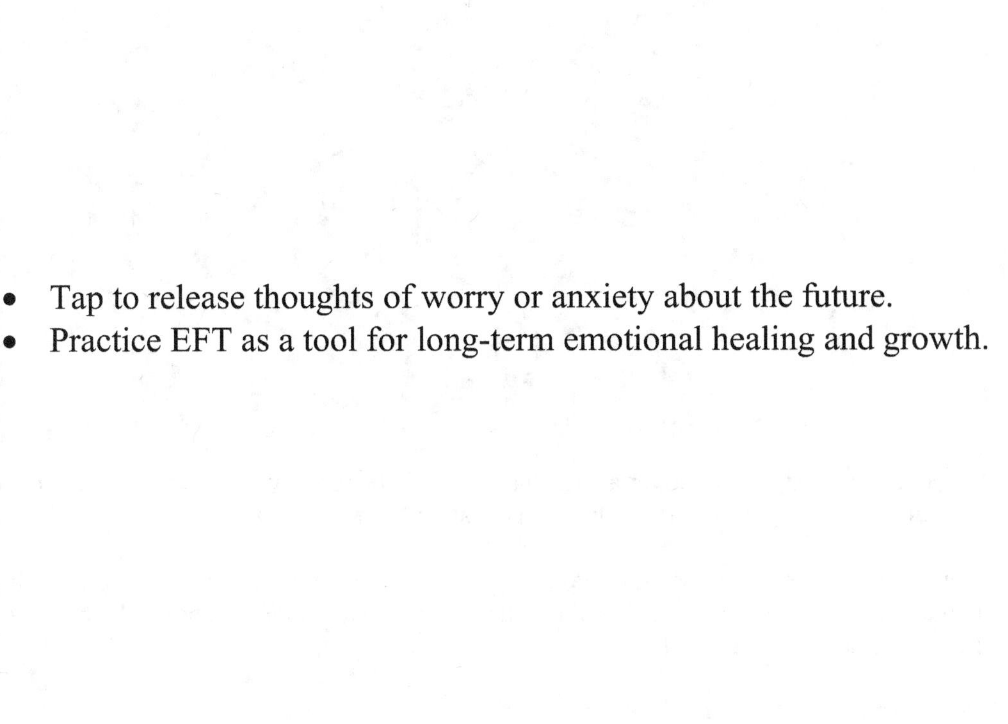

- Tap to release thoughts of worry or anxiety about the future.
- Practice EFT as a tool for long-term emotional healing and growth.

Have Questions / Comments?

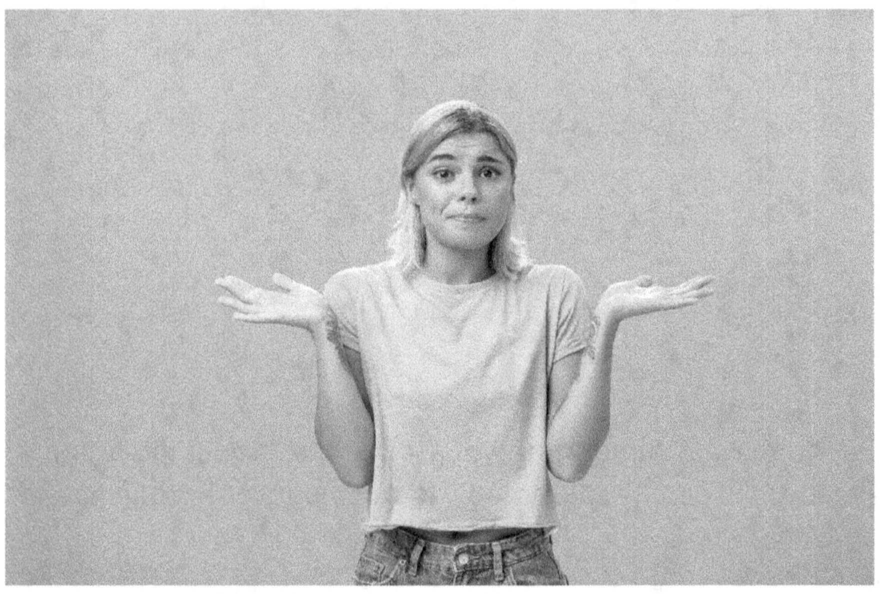

This book was designed to cover as much as possible but I know I have probably missed something, or some new amazing discovery that has just come out.

If you notice something missing or have a question that I failed to answer, please get in touch and let me know. If I can, I will email you an answer and also update the book so others can also benefit from it.

Thanks For Being Awesome :)

Submit Your Questions / Comments At:

https://questions.xspurts.com

Get Another Book Free

We love writing and have produced a huge number of books.

For being one of our amazing readers, we would love to offer you another book we have created, 100% free.

To claim this limited time special offer, simply go to the site below and enter your name and email address.

You will then receive one of my great books, direct to your email account, 100% free!

https://free.xspurts.com

9 798340 288028